The Art of LOVE-MAKING

The Art of LOVE-MAKING

An Illustrated

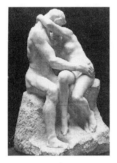

Tribute

James A. Haught

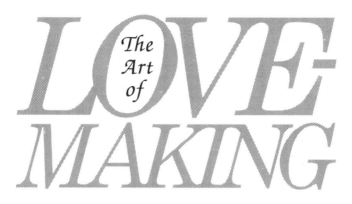

With an Introduction by
Russell C. Vannoy

PROMETHEUS BOOKS
Buffalo, New York

Published 1992 by Prometheus Books

96 95 94 93 92   5 4 3 2 1

Library of Congress Cataloging-in-Publication Data

Haught, James A.
    The art of lovemaking : an illustrated tribute / James A. Haught.
With an introduction by Russell C. Vannoy.
        p.   cm.
    Includes index.
    ISBN 0-87975-740-X (cloth : alk paper)
    1. Erotica. 2. Esthetics. 3. Art—Philosophy. 4. Love in Art.
I. Title.
HQ460.H38   1992
306.7—dc20   92-29847
                                                                    CIP

Printed in the United States of America on acid-free paper.

CONTENTS

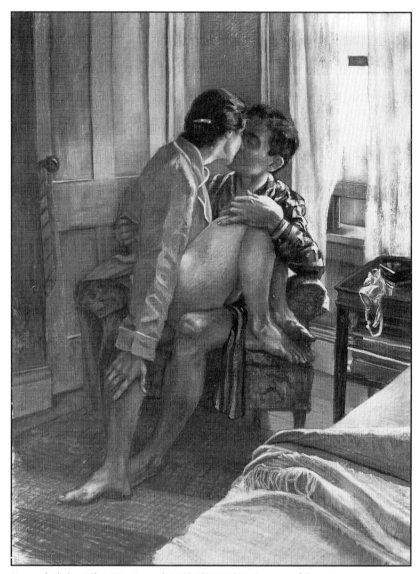

Sigmund Abeles. "Their Kiss," pastel, 1989 (68″ × 48″). Courtesy of the artist.

INTRODUCTION

SEX, ART, AND BEAUTY

The editor of this beautiful collection of erotica claims that sex is "healthy, natural, wholesome, joyful, romantic, tender, fulfilling, and utterly wonderful." In the age of AIDS, this viewpoint, if true, surely comes as a welcome reassurance. To build an enduring philosophy of sex around a plague is also quite short-sighted; for when the plague is over, a cynical philosophy is bereft of that support. Furthermore, if these paintings, statues, and drawings do capture the essence of sex, James Haught is right and modern-day puritans like the Moral Majority and certain feminists are dead wrong. Hardly anyone today would, of course, say that *all* sex is dirty or evil. When Andrea Dworkin in her book, *Intercourse*, claims that all genital penetration, consensual or not, is a violation of the boundaries of a woman' s body, she feels that she is stating the truth as much as Haught does. But when a feminist says that all traditional genital sex is rape, the "is" is linked to the claim that sex *ought* to be viewed differently. This means sex that is free of dominance and submission, sex that is based on mutuality and reciprocity, and sex that is sensuous rather than genital.

The claim that genital sex *inherently* violates mutuality and

7

reciprocity (as opposed to contingent facts about patriarchy) is, however, surely only a personal truth for Dworkin and her followers. Indeed, some of the pictures contained in this volume do depict politically incorrect male-on-top genital sex. Yet even here what the artist portrays seems to combine the sensuous and the passionate in an ethereal way that contradicts the feminist attack on genital sex as a three-minute missionary-position ejaculation service that leaves women sexually unfulfilled and ruthlessly objectified by male dominance. Are we being seduced and misled by art (as Plato feared), or does art reveal a deeper truth that contradicts feminist theory?

Haught's philosophy of the inherent beauty of sex is derived from eighteenth-century Romanticism. In much less romantic form the idea of the goodness of sex lives on in the writings of Alfred Kinsey, Masters & Johnson, Hugh Hefner, and Shere Hite in this century. But what if sex isn't always so beautiful? Are concepts like sexual immorality or sexual perversity contradictions in terms? (They would be if sex were intrinsically good.) It is no use saying that sexual immorality is merely a misuse of something good; for evil deeds can be, for some, quite sexy just because they are evil. Or what about a perversely beautiful painting of the rape of the Sabine women? Note that Haught says that sex *is* beautiful, not merely that it can be or ought to be beautiful. The "is" might seem to be as dogmatic as Dworkin's "is not." Once again, however, the "is beautiful" for a romantic really means "can be beautiful" if we only remove the dirty lenses society has given us through which we view nature and sex. Were sex seen in its natural purity, then it would cease to be used to dirty, hurt, or humiliate others. Although Haught does not say this, it is quite compatible with his optimistic concept of sex. A cynic about sex would, of course, hold that any claims about dirty minds abusing the beauty of sex are analogous to the NRA's view that people and not guns are responsible for murder.

The naturalist has another line of attack, however. He can simply say that sex which isn't wonderful (that of the Marquis de Sade or Jeffrey Dahmer) isn't really sex at all. For if sex is beautiful and it is made into something ugly, then it can't really be sex if beauty is one of its essential qualities. (The "beauty" aspect for romantics is commonly defined as expressing love, whereas Hugh Hefner's hedonism defined sex as beautiful just by itself.) But if ugly sex is no longer sex, then what is it? The familiar reply is that it is now merely an act of violence or a power trip. The view that it's either sex *or* else it's violence is really quite a remarkable dualism. Why, for example, should anyone worry about aborting a pregnancy caused by rape if sex wasn't somehow involved? Or why is rape viewed as a uniquely vicious and degrading form of assault that is quite different from being hit in the head and perhaps being damaged more severely in a physical sense? Perhaps, however, the rape-isn't-sex claim is merely a way of saying that violent sex is only a *means* of exercising power over others and is not the motive. (Note that sex couldn't even be a secondary motive in rape since sex is, by definition, held to be utterly beautiful.) Yet using sex as a means to power wouldn't mean that it ceases to be sex, any more than money would cease to be money were it used for the same reason.

Indeed, sex as a means to an end is quite different from, say, using a condom as a means of preventing disease and (hopefully) forgetting it is even there. For if sex is a means of exercising power, it must be powerful itself; nor can it be forgotten in the way a condom might be ignored. But then the means and the goal become interwired, power becomes eroticized, and sex and power have at least equal status if they can be distinguished at all. In pornographic films depicting violence, the rapist begins with a desire to degrade his victim. But as the scene progresses, he invariably finds himself saying (sometimes in an almost pleading way), "You like it, don't you? You know you do, honey." The lust for power has seemingly changed to language that is often found in normal sex.

Here the sexual optimist could say that the rapist is, in a perverse way, seeking the reciprocity that marks the beauty of sex in its normal forms, and that power is merely a means of doing what he cannot achieve consensually. Were he able to show this, the naturalist wouldn't have to fall back on the claim that sexual violence isn't really sexual in order to protect his claim that sex is inherently beautiful. Yet a sexual pessimist could also say that what the rapist finds erotic is inflicting pleasure on someone, perversely compelling her to enjoy at the sensory level what she rationally feels is utterly abominable. Which view is right is impossible to decide here. One is, however, surely tempted to say that claims about whether sex is inherently beautiful or ugly are prescriptive rather than descriptive.

Indeed, an existentialist would hold (correctly, I think) that neither nature nor sex have any inherent value; they are simply brute facts. It is only when we make authentic choices that are genuinely our own about what to do with sex that values come into play. An orgasm, of course, might seem to be a brute fact which is inherently valuable because it overwhelms us with ecstasy. Yet we can also choose to evaluate the facticity of an

orgasm in divergent ways—as an out-of-body religious experience which is also the ultimate bodily experience; as a cheap
thrill; as *le petit mort*; as an annoying attack on our rationality; or,
ambivalently, as being like fireworks that gloriously light up the
sky, but whose explosion is also their destruction, leaving us in
the darkness from whence we came. Or one could say that fireworks and orgasms provide a timeless experience in which there
is no "before" or "after." How one feels afterward is simply
irrelevant to what counts—the transcendent experience itself.

A naturalist sexologist would, of course, find most of these
choices to be a sign of one's hang-ups about sexual pleasure and
that therapy is in order. Yet it does seem quite possible for a
normal person to choose to view sexual ecstasy with either total
surrender or ambivalence. To relish the climax of a play without
reservations or to realize that its power also spells the end of a
beautiful two-hour performance are surely both very human
options.

Or one person may choose to enjoy sex with love and
another choose to divorce sex from love. Is the latter choice
unhealthy, as many would claim? The romantic would view love
between two persons as a fascinating and charming paradox of
two separate persons who become one, but who also retain
their individuality. For him or her, sex with love is thereby
saved in the *only* way possible from cold, mechanistic, egocentric anonymity. Yet the nonromantic might choose to view the
paradox of two separate persons who also supposedly merge as
an unresolvable and agonizing dilemma if he or she is to be
intellectually honest. Furthermore, sex can be a loving, generous
act even if it is between strangers. Neither point of view seems
to be absolutely right for everyone. Hence the existentialists' dis-

11

taste for the view that there is one and only one "healthy" attitude toward sex.

Haught's philosophy, as I noted above, is classic Romantic naturalism. It rejects the dour conservative claim that sex as sex is a dark, Dionysian force that destroys our Apollonian self-control and rationality. The comedian George Carlin once asked, "What does cocaine feel like? It feels like more cocaine." This is the conservative view of sex, one that liberals sometimes share when they refer to the supposed effects of adult sex on a child. (Interestingly, Freud, a villain to conservatives, had the same demonic view of the libido.) For the conservative, sex must be domesticated and made useful around the house as an expression of married love and as a natural way of making babies.

For the conservative, something like true homosexuality (as opposed to merely frustrated or frightened heterosexuality) is a contradiction since sex, love, marriage, and children are said to be *conceptually* linked. Even if one could show that there were perverse pleasures, the conservative would still insist that perverse happiness is a contradiction. For this combination of sex and traditional family is supposedly ordained by God or Nature as the *only* form of sexual happiness possible. Unlike the existentialist who feels we can choose among sex or marriage or love or children or any combination of these (or none at all), the conservative believes that Nature's truth is self-evident and that choice might only lead one astray. Hence the traditional desire to rigidly regulate sex, something that should actually be unnecessary if the conservative view is as obviously true and natural as it claims.

Interestingly, the romantic reaction to conservative sexual

philosophy leaves intact certain traditions, now baptized in the concept of benign, beautiful naturalness. There is the claim that men and women are "meant" for each other. This view, however, leaves women with no option except to be attached to a man. To be sure, a romantic male does put his Fair Lady on a pedestal to be worshiped as a goddess. Yet this prevents him from seeing her as a person. Indeed, being on a pedestal is lonely and quite stressful in maintaining the illusion of perfection needed to stimulate the male's delicious fantasies. (Witness Princess Diana's problems as a goddess for the public.)

The claim that men and women are "meant" for each other also makes even the existence of homosexuality quite problematic. Why did the Romantic philosophy of smashing sterile constricting tradition with the purity of passion and a return to nature neglect smashing a certain ambivalent kind of sexism and homophobia? Was the Romantics' concept of nature too narrow? Did they fail to realize that their own passions may have been in part social constructs that reason (had they taken reason seriously) could have ferreted out?

Or was it because whatever provides one with an ecstatic experience is seen as being infinitely superior to anything else? (Hence the problem of the woman on the pedestal.) That is, perhaps the problem lies in the nature of Romantic ecstasy itself. If I am a heterosexual and have been, as it were, to the mountain top of passion, don't I conclude not just that this woman and I are meant for each other, but that *men and women* are meant for each other? Since romantics view themselves as individualists, it may seem puzzling that the fact that Sue and I love each other would lead to an unwarranted generalization about men and women as a whole. Yet when one is lifted out of oneself in romantic ecstasy and made one with all of nature, there is nothing that is merely true "for us." We are the world, or at least we have what everyone would ideally like to have— heterosexual love. Hence: "Men and women are meant for each other."

Those down in the valley who haven't climbed to my peak experience are simply viewed as being unaware of the truth that ecstasy reveals. I may tolerate the poor souls in the valley or I may even sincerely fight for the civil rights of sexual minorities. Yet I can never accept their pleasures as being equal to mine in terms of their passionate intensity. Romantics of other sexual orientations that disagree with mine also feel the same way about their ecstasy. In this respect, sex is something like religion: One can be as ecumenical as one likes, but no true believer ever thinks that other religions reveal the truth quite like one's own. Within this framework, perpetual conflict (sometimes overt, sometimes very subtle) is assured.

Although romantics do not much identify sex with marriage and children, they do have, as it were, a religion of romantic love. In one way it is curiously conservative about sex. This "religion" often seems to despise sex unless it can serve a further goal, i.e., sex as a vehicle for expressing love. To use a food analogy, it is as if they found black coffee (plain sex) to be bitter and can enjoy it only when it is sweetened with lots of cream and sugar, i.e., love. Perhaps the reader of this book can discern his or her preferences by seeing which of the sensuously erotic pictures appeal most.

Note, however, that the preceding coffee analogy does not apply to those who do enjoy plain sex, but rather to those who have the additive view that combining two types of passion, sex

14

and love, is better than having just one. The additive view does, however, presuppose that romantic sensuousness (kissing, caressing) and raw genital passion are quite compatible. Yet lusty genital sex (or any form of sex leading to orgasm) makes it very difficult to think of romance; consciousness identifies with the body with such a ferocious intensity that the tenderness of kissing and caressing that expresses love is utterly left behind in the realm of "foreplay" so loved by romantics. Indeed, at the moment of orgasm, one can't express anything to anybody since one is completely absorbed in one's own ecstatic experience. The lover may be delighted to see the beloved's orgasm as proof of his ability to please his beloved; yet he also feels curiously alone when the beloved clenches her fist, closes her eyes, and shakes uncontrollably. One suspects that romantics would prefer to limit sex to foreplay; yet caressing and kissing also notoriously stimulate the body in quite a different direction. One suspects that the attempt to combine sex and love is a con-tradictory ideal, a view romantics would vigorously reject.

Haught's charming collection of paintings and drawings does appear to depict sex-positive acts. Yet even these seemingly innocent works of art are anathema to the utilitarian conserva-tive—ironically, perhaps even more so than straightforward por-nography. For erotica compels us to take an esthetic attitude toward sex, in the way that the nude compels us to look at the naked in quite a different way. The esthetic attitude is com-monly described as a kind of disinterested contemplation of an object or an act for its own sake. We stand transfixed by the sheer beauty (or even ugliness) of something which we find utterly fascinating and wholly absorbing. Whatever might dis-turb this esthetic fixation is rigidly excluded.

This would seemingly make Haught's collection quite different from pornography, which is anything but disinterested. Pornography is ordinarily purchased for a quite self-interested, utilitarian motive—to become sexually aroused. But the conservative is suspicious of all this. Doesn't erotica somehow make sexual enjoyment beautiful by transforming it into art, whereas pornography supposedly reveals sex in all its ugliness and thus perversely confirms the conservative view? Nor is disinterested contemplation ever quite *that* disinterested when sex is the subject matter of art. For a carefully sculpted nude may be far more erotic than a warts-and-all naked person.

Erotica is legally protected because of its esthetic value and because it is assumed that the cooler esthetic contemplation of form dampens the sexual arousal produced by the content. A sociological reason may be that those who are sufficiently "refined" to find a nude sexually interesting are also believed to be capable of controlling their passions. The supposedly lower orders who buy pornography are viewed quite differently.

But the conservative still has doubts about all this. Erotica is, for him, perverse because it is both cool and hot, both beautiful and obscene. Ambivalence is a threat to his orderly "straight" world and cannot be tolerated. Even worse, if sex can be *viewed* esthetically or contemplated for its own sake, why can't it then be *engaged* in for its own sake? Doesn't the mixing of the esthetic and the sexual mean that the former will ultimately lead to the latter, given the power of any sexual content? While this doesn't mean that one will caress a statue, it does mean that one may desire to caress a statuesque person and enjoy him or her sexually even when there are no thoughts of love, marriage, reproduction, or perhaps even traditional genital sex.

Indeed, pornography may seem to be less of a threat to the conservative's world: it is what it is, and is not nearly so subversively duplicitous as erotica. For the conservative, pornography is a marvelous lesson in what sex enjoyed for its own sake really is—dirty and disgusting. And it is—he thinks—produced by sexual radicals who love to wallow in the dirt he despises. The pornographer is thus as essential to the conservative as the Communists were to right-wing politicians—a menace that kept their movement united and strong by having an enemy to fight.

There is irony aplenty in all this, but the contradictions are not nearly as bothersome as an artist's making sex as sex something beautiful to behold. This is a contradiction for the conservative; yet the artist has done it. It-can't-be-but-yet-it-is is the ultimate dizzying thought when it goes to the very heart of one's philosophy. The producer of erotica is thus not so much seen as someone who deviates from an established norm as one who willfully causes us to feel contradictory states of mind, by making what is necessarily ugly also to be somehow beautiful. The conservative is thus ultimately more threatened by what he views as *perversity* than he is by straightforward perversion.

The conservative, however, is right on one point: Sex and art do have the power to disorder our cherished identities and ordinary views about what is true, good, and beautiful. When we are not sexually aroused, many of the sexual positions depicted in this volume may seem grotesque or laughable. When we are sexually excited, however, these same positions become curiously beautiful, perhaps because we associate them with beautifully passionate experiences.

Is it possible to comprehend sex? Conservatives would compare sex with alcohol. Like cocaine, alcohol always tastes like more alcohol. Thus sex, unless carefully controlled, becomes addictive, destroys one's reason and social constraints, and could plunge the world into chaos were it not carefully regulated. A few sips of wine before dinner is the conservative analogue to domesticated sex. Naturalists who view sex more benignly, however, often use a food metaphor: sex is a wholesome, healthy appetite like savoring a fine meal (romantic sex). Or it is like a quick stop at Burger King simply to quell hunger pangs (promiscuous, anonymous sex). Adultery would be analogous to a stranger's taking one's beloved out to dinner, masturbation would be eating alone, and rape would be like force-feeding someone. Although the analogy is often used in a non-judgmental way, e.g., being straight or gay is like choosing between apples and oranges, it is also often quite judgmental. Note the familiar invidious comparison of sexual love with anonymous sex: the latter is actually about novelty and adventure rather than simply releasing sexual tensions. And it is as selective as the appetite of those who dine at a swank restaurant.

The gustatory analogy, however, fails in a deeper way. Why do we prefer living flesh to dead meat, however tasty a steak may be? One answer would be that we want to sexually communicate various feelings, attitudes, and emotions with another person. (Masturbation, therefore, would be like communicating with oneself in a diary.) Another answer is that we want both to receive and give sensory experiences: I am aroused by another's arousal, which further arouses me and further arouses another, and so forth.

The food analogy is also inapt as a way of talking about sexual love. Eating something is a rather egocentric desire to completely consume it, to make it part of one's being. If, however, both lovers desire to absorb each other, conflict ensues when each wants to possess the other. What romantic love wants is a kind of merging of two identities, a surrender of each to the other. If sex is simply like eating something, it could not serve as an expression of love. Merely sharing a meal is not, of course, egocentric; but the sharing of two bodies in sexual love has a much more complex dynamic that requires a more subtle analogy. A skeptic could, of course, argue that sex *is* like eating, and too bad for sexual love; for sex is so different from love that it can't possibly express it. Interestingly, some advocates of sexual love also claim that sex by itself is egocentric and cold. But if plain sex is inherently ugly, how does it remain sex when it expresses love, or how could it ever express love to begin with? If, on the other hand, sex and love are sufficiently similar that sex could express love, the supposedly absolute superiority of sexual love to plain sex disappears. Indeed, the sexual organs are neither egocentric nor altrustic; persons are. And persons can be generous, whether or not they are in love.

Another analogy is that of recreation, popularized by Hugh Hefner in the *Playboy* philosophy. Recreational sex is supposed to be good, clean, innocent fun, although this is not exactly what the early Romantic had in mind in proclaiming the beauty of sex. Sexual intercourse is thus like playing tennis; masturbation is like jogging alone; and prostitution would be like professional athletics. Although adultery would resemble one's beloved playing tennis with a stranger, it is not so clear that this would be viewed with the horror one often feels about sexual infidelity.

Indeed, tennis and other games have a winner and a loser, hardly an apt way to describe fully consensual sex. Perhaps one could avoid the winner-loser problem by comparing sex to two persons jogging side by side for the fun of it or "roughhousing," i.e., playfully poking each other. Yet sex sometimes "gets serious," as lovers say when they are trying to communicate an important emotion like love. Can the recreation analogy capture this? When roughhousing (or even jogging together) gets serious, it does turn into a contest (wrestling or racing) with a winner and a loser. Once again the analogy violates the notion of fully consensual sexual acts. Nor is the picture of recreation (and thus of sex) as good clean fun quite accurate. Killing endangered species of wildlife for sport is no more lovely than sadistic sex. Indeed, the eating analogy is not always benign either: the most perfect example of eroticized eating was Jeffrey Dahmer's cannibalism.

Since this is a book of erotica, perhaps one should describe sex in terms of an art form. My choice is the dance. Unlike the eating analogy, it is something that occurs between persons who are not thereby consumed in the process. Dancing can, like recreational sex, be done for fun; yet it can also "get serious," e.g., when disco dancing is interrupted for a bit of slow-dancing for-lovers-only in a darkened hall. Unlike games, however, dance does not invariably turn into a contest between the two partners, with a winner and a loser, when this shift of mood occurs. Were one or both partners in a wild headbangers' dance at a Heavy Metal concert actually to *intend* to cause a concussion, it would no longer be a dance. (The sexual analogue of this is found in extreme forms of consensual sadomasochism.) In exceptional cases, dancing might be demonic: a tribal war dance is an example. And dance can upset one's everyday identity, as when the austere professor, tired of his rationality, finds himself with a desire to boogie to rap music.

The most artistic dance form, the ballet, also reflects a central philosophical debate about what sex should be. Some prefer an expansionist account in which sex must be conjoined with "significance" and "meaning" in terms of being linked to the expression of a wide range of emotions through body language; or sex must be conjoined with "family values." The same must be true for ballet, some argue. Conservatives adore the *Nutcracker Suite* since it tugs at the heartstrings, tells a story, and requires that both sexes be part of the performance; minimalists (like myself), however, view the richness of *Nutcracker* as being more analogous to that of a big hot fudge sundae. Minimalist ballet emphasizes spontaneous movements, done quite sparingly, that allow one to focus on the pure beauty of the forms of bodies in motion. So it is with plain sex as well, a view that is considered shallow and the perverse triumph of style over substance by expansionists. When the controversy over sexual philosophies is expressed in terms of divergent tastes about ballet, a live-and-let-live truce is surely warranted.

Where does this beautiful book of erotica stand in relation to the dance metaphor? One could say that erotica's depiction of "classy" sex relates to ordinary sex in the way that ballet is comparable to the two-step. However, that would seem to turn the art of lovemaking in its most elegant form into a highly specialized skilled performance. We ordinary mortals could only gape at it in wonder and admiration, but never hope to emulate it. Yet the lived experience of the ordinary dancer and a ballerina may have interesting structural similarities. When one has a compatible, interesting, adept partner or partners, the square dancer can feel as ecstatic and godlike as Nureyev. If so, then

21

couldn't the "square" lover feel like Romeo, even if he looks like a dolt to someone who isn't sharing his experience?

No one would, of course, buy a book like this if all it did was show Edith and Archie Bunker making love. So what? In erotic reality, the ordinary can become extraordinary for those who surrender to its charms. Although seemingly elitist, what erotica captures in art is the transcendence in which we can all partake when we have the opportunity for such an experience. An epiphany is an epiphany, even if what Archie and Edith share would seem crude to Romeo and Juliet. Things like sexism, puritanism, homophobia, ageism, and narrow concepts about the body beautiful must, of course, be overcome before the opportunity for erotic ecstasy is available to everyone. Perhaps the dance metaphor points the way: Square dancing cares little about the body beautiful, age, or social class; disco dancing is gender-neutral and non-homophobic; and even the ballet is available to anyone who has the talent to meet its demands. And dancing generally honors the feminist ideals of nonhierarchical mutuality and reciprocity in sex. What Haught's extraordinary collection has given us, then, is ecstasy captured in artistic form, an ecstasy that could perhaps be available to everyone if only the world had dance fever and viewed sex accordingly. Read, view, and enjoy the pages that follow.

Russell C. Vannoy

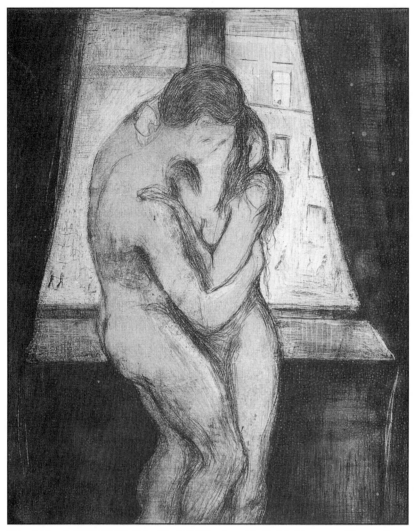

Edvard Munch (1869–1944). "The Kiss" (1895). Copyright © Oslo Kommunes Kunstamlinger.
By permission of the Munch-Museet, Oslo.

SEX IS BEAUTIFUL

W hy do men and women everywhere crave to unite in lovemaking?

In Plato's *Symposium*, one of the debaters, the comic poet Aristophanes, gave this answer: humans once were bizarre, eight-limbed creatures, but Zeus split them into halves, male and female. Ever since, the sundered pairs have felt a compulsion to rejoin. This urge, he said, is "the love which restores us to our ancient state by attempting to weld two beings into one and heal the wounds which humanity suffered."

Modern science has other explanations. Yet Aristophanes was right on one point: sex can heal the wounds of life, giving couples inner peace. It generates contentment and commitment, love and laughter—joys added like jewels to the biological act of reproduction.

This book is rooted in the view that sex is healthy, natural, wholesome, joyful, romantic, tender, fulfilling, and utterly wonderful. Moreover, a fascinating beauty exists when a man and woman entwine in the primal union. Artists and poets of many centuries have expressed it. Their works are presented here to illustrate the book's theme that sex is beautiful.

And yet, perversely, some people see ugliness. Western taboos tinge sex with shame, making it a "dirty" topic to be censored and hidden. Bodies are deemed obscene.

How did guilt attach to sex? Some anthropologists say it was because the genitals are near the excretory parts of the body. Others add that male supremacy was a factor. Masters who kept women as possessions needed to hide the females' charms under garments, lest other males be tempted to trespass upon the owners' property. Thus concealment became customary. Later, Western religions codified shame.

The global record of art tells the sexual story of past cultures—and also reveals ploys which artists used to circumvent strictures of their times. The drawings, carvings, and paintings in this book recount this human chronicle.

In classical Greece, sex was portrayed without guilt. Painted vases and bowls depicted lovers cavorting. As the Greeks colonized the Mediterranean basin and traded with foreign peoples, the ceramic trade expanded widely. Today, Greek pottery is found in various far-flung archeological excavations.

After the Romans captured Greek colonies in the Italian peninsula, then took Greece itself, they adopted Greek art, including conventionalized portrayals of lovers. By the 1st century B.C.E., Romans were celebrating sex in erotic wall frescoes, marble carvings, sculpted pottery, mirror cases, and the like.

Then religion brought a dozen centuries of suppression. Judaism had always criminalized much of sex, decreeing death for unmarried lovers. Christianity intensified the taboo. Church founders reviled sex; Tertullian, for example, recommended that all women should be veiled. Origen reportedly castrated himself to elude temptation. According to Augustine, sex was the vehicle through which Eve's original sin was passed from generation to generation. Pope Gregory I wrote that "sexual pleasure can never be without sin." The Age of Faith banished erotic imagery, except for moralistic pictures of punished sinners or the temptation of Adam and Eve.

Meanwhile, Asia was spared this guilt. Sex was portrayed without shame in India, China, and Japan. Lovemaking is natural to Hindus, so they deemed it appropriate for their many gods and goddesses. Carvers of India's great temples 900 years ago filled them with copulating deities. In the Tantric branch of the faith, sex was performed as a religious ritual. China and Japan developed a tradition of sexual drawings and prints, such as "pillow books" given to newlyweds to show them the ways of love.

In the West, the flowering of the Renaissance finally enabled sex to reappear—in guises acceptable to the church. Artists revived Greek and Roman mythology, teeming with nude nymphs and goddesses frolicking with gods and satyrs. By pretending that the couples they displayed weren't real people, painters and sculptors eluded censure. Art historian Bradley Smith notes that the ancient deities became "established devices for portraying naked human passions and unclothed human bodies."

Also, subterranean erotica circulated among the privileged elite (including some within the church). For example, Raphael's favorite pupil, Giulio Romano (1499–1546), painted a dozen copulating couples in various positions—allegedly at the request of worldly Pope Leo X. Engraver Marcantonio Raimondi reproduced the scenes on copper plates and they were printed with sonnets in a clandestine book, I Modi (the modes of lovemaking). After Leo's death, puritanical Pope Clement VII jailed Raimondi, but Giulio had moved to Mantua, and thus escaped. His "postures" have been recopied ever since.

In ensuing centuries, artists continued using mythological or allegorical figures, often surrounding nude couples with cupids. Slowly, real human sex began appearing in locales where church pressure subsided. Dutch master Rembrandt van Rijn (1606–

1669) depicted an enraptured bourgeois couple in bed in an etching titled "Ledikant" or "Lit à la Francaise."

By the late 19th century, lovers were legitimate in art—but censorship backlashes were common. Sculptor Auguste Rodin created his renowned "The Kiss" in the 1890s. Yet two decades later, Viennese artist Egon Schiele was jailed for making erotic sketches. The struggle between candor and prudery is endless, even though the sexual revoltuion has kept the latter in retreat.

After World War II, Supreme Court rulings in America established what has been called "the right to see." A landmark 1973 decision ruled that depictions of "ultimate sexual acts" can be banned only if they're patently offensive, without social value, and contrary to community standards. (The ruling sometimes elicits amused speculation about what constitutes an ultimate sexual act. Lovers in a rubber raft going over Niagara Falls? A couple atop the Eiffel Tower in a lightning storm? Two elephants in a china shop?)

Despite the court breakthroughs, hundreds of fundamentalist groups around America still clamor for laws against "filth," and conservative politicians support them. Some feminists have joined the cause but for different reasons, contending that sexual portrayals degrade women.

But the art in this book refutes them all. It demonstrates that sex need not be "dirty." It also repudiates the pornographers who reduce all sex to the level of the crude and vulgar. Obviously, the artists—from the ancient Greeks to 1990s American painters—have seen lovers as affectionate equals, sharing joy. What sort of person is repelled by that?

The book is intended for the private enjoyment of couples, to reinforce all that is good in their feelings for each other.

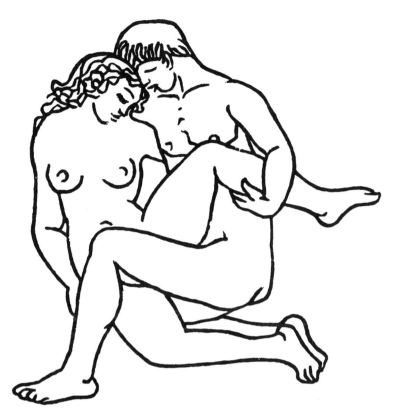

Aristide Maillol (1861–1944). Woodcut illustration for the *Odes* of Horace. © 1992 ARS, N.Y./SPADEM, Paris.

Come, let us take our fill of love until the morning; let us solace ourselves with loves.

—Proverbs 7

Remove that hindering robe; take down your hair; let naked limbs be locked with naked limbs. . . . Now breast to breast, mouth into mouth, till all is plunged into the depths, and we lie still.

—Meleager, *The Greek Anthology*, 2nd century B.C.

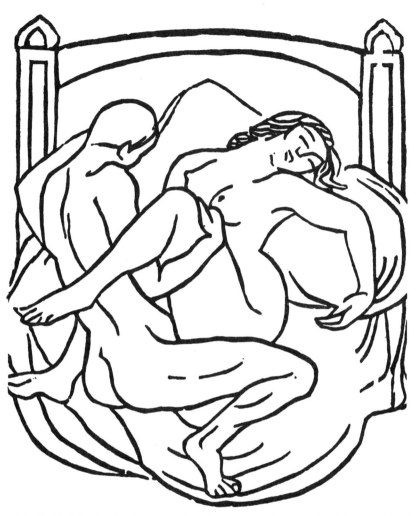

Aristide Maillol. Woodcut illustration for *Chansons pour Elle* (1939), Bibliothèque Nationale.
© 1992 ARS, N.Y./SPADEM, Paris.

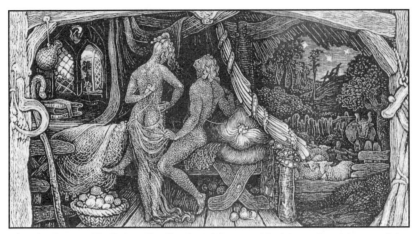

Edward Calvert (1799–1883). "The Chamber Idyll," print. The Metropolitan Museum of Art, Harris Brisbane Dick Fund, 1931. (31.87.41). The Metropolitan Museum of Art.

Sex appeal is the keynote of our civilization.
        —Henri Bergson (1859–1941), *Creative Evolution*

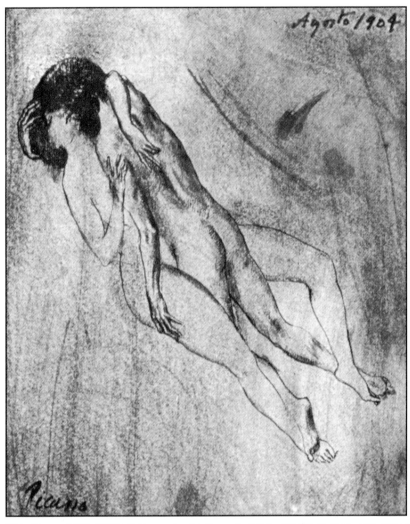

Pablo Picasso (1881–1973). Self-portrait with Fernande Olivier (1904). © 1992 ARS, N.Y./ SPADEM, Paris.

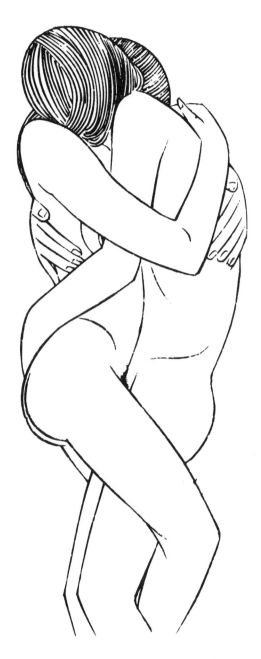

Eric Gill (1882–1940). "Lovers," wood engraving. Victoria and Albert Museum/Art Resource, N.Y.

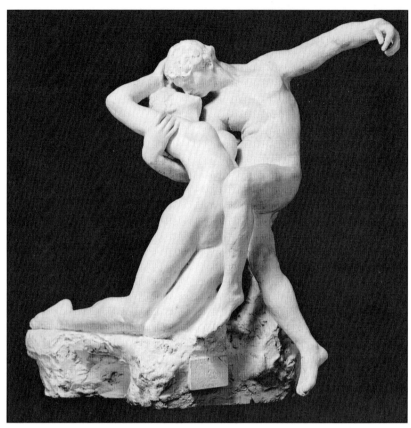

Auguste Rodin (1840–1917). "Eternal Springtime," plaster group (1884). Philadelphia Museum. Given by Paul Rosenberg.

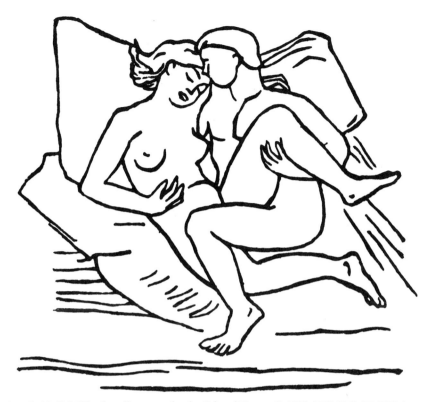

Aristide Maillol. Woodcut illustration for the *Odes* of Horace. © 1992 ARS, N.Y./SPADEM, Paris.

I lie all melting in her charms
And fast locked up within her legs and arms.
 —John Sheffield (1648–1721), "The Happy Night"

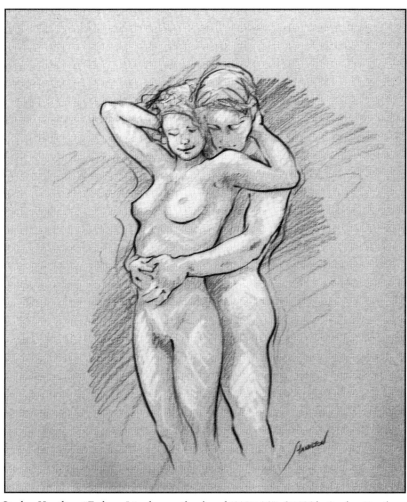

Stephen Hamilton. "Embrace I," color pencil on board (11" × 14"). © 1990 by Stephen Hamilton. Courtesy of the artist.

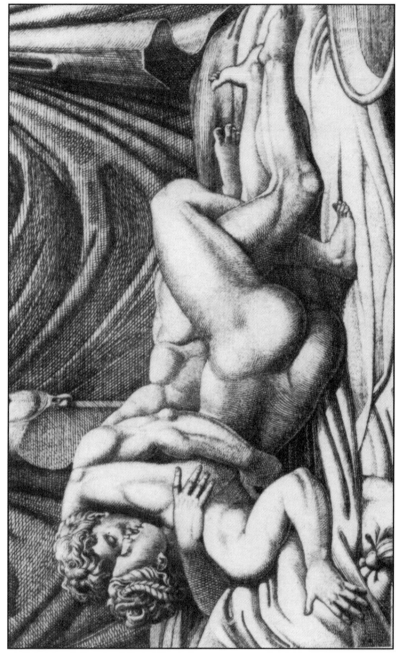

Drawing by Giulio Romano (1499–1546), engraved by Marcantonio Raimondi (1480–1534) for *I Modi*, a clandestine book showing the modes, or positions, of lovemaking.

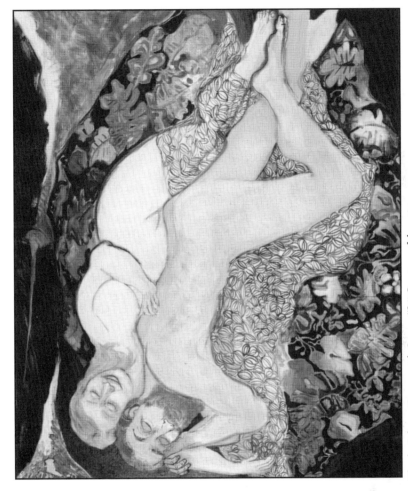

Phoebe Palmer. "Lovers with Covers #2." Courtesy of the artist.

41

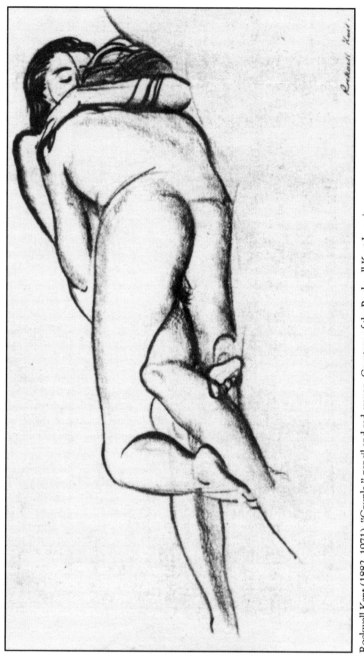

Rockwell Kent (1882–1971). "Couple," pencil and red crayon. Courtesy of the Rockwell Kent Legacies.

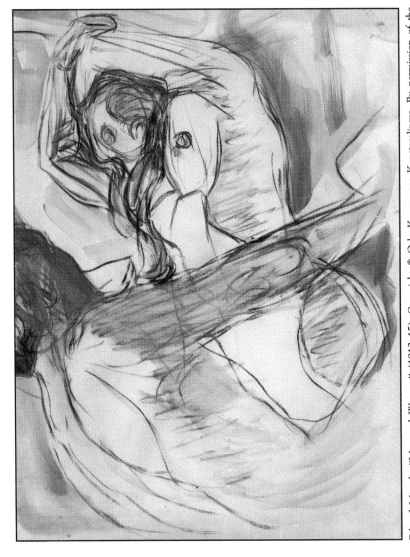

Edvard Munch. "Man and Woman" (1912–15). Copyright © Oslo Kommunes Kunstamlinger. By permission of the Munch-Museet, Oslo.

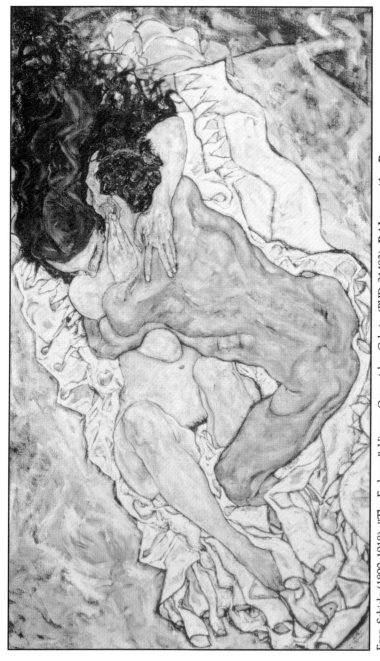

Egon Schiele (1890–1918). "The Embrace." Vienna: Osterreiches Galerie. (PHD 21483). **Bridgeman/Art Resource, New York.**

44

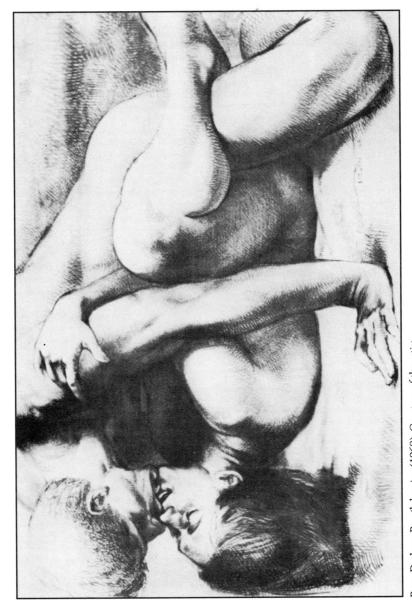

Betty Dodson. Pencil drawing (1968). Courtesy of the artist.

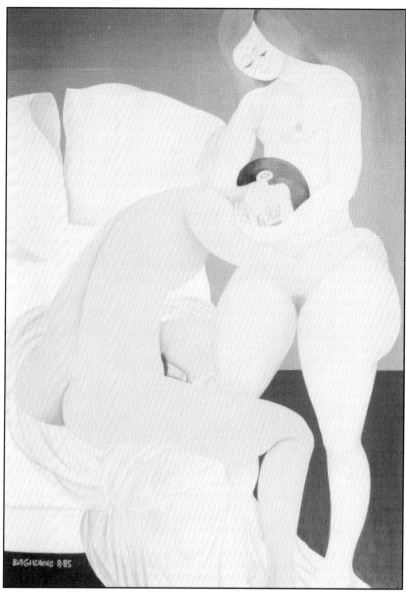

Bill Giacalone. "Lovers," acrylic (46″ × 66″). Courtesy of the artist.

46

Clasping and twining
And panting and wishing
And sighing and kissing
And sighing and kissing so close.
　　　　—John Dryden (1631–1700), "Sylvia, the Fair"

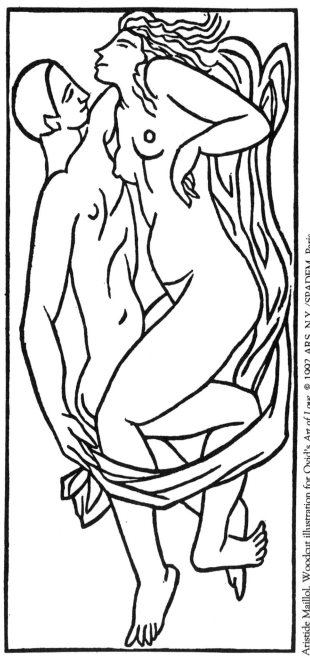

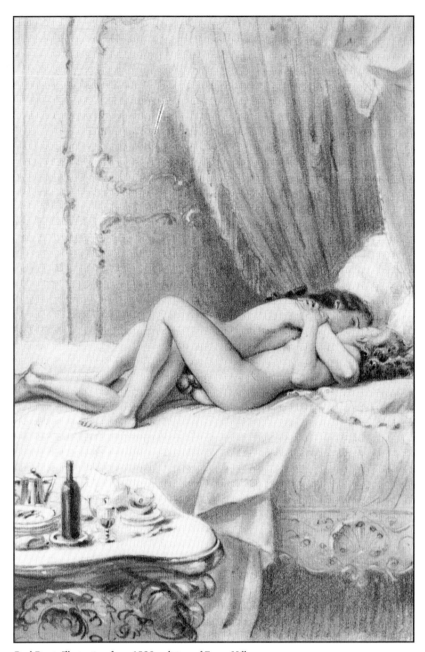

Paul Becat. Illustration for a 1930s edition of *Fanny Hill*.

MULTITUDES, MULTITUDES

Look out over a city at night.
   Picture in your mind, throughout that glimmering ocean, the hundreds, perhaps *thousands*, of couples making love—in dimmed homes, apartments, hotel rooms, parked cars, even boats. Some on office couches, park benches, or sleeping bags on rooftops.

Teenagers, middle-agers, affluent, poor, whites, blacks, Orientals, Hispanics—everywhere in intimate privacy, two by two, obeying the universal law of nature.

And yet, the tableau is invisible. The observable world—scurrying crowds, noisy traffic, flashing lights, busy theaters and restaurants—is oblivious to the drama occurring behind countless doors. Even the secluded lovers are unaware of their unseen counterparts everywhere in the night.

Lovemaking is all-encompassing. Its magic applies to everyone. As the poet Joseph Addison put it, couples of every sort "sink in the soft captivity together."

Think of the numbers: Researchers say American couples have intercourse, on average, about one night in three. The 1990 census counted 60 million married pairs, while millions of others live together or date steadily. So, on any night, from the boroughs of New York to the teeming Los Angeles suburbs and all points between, perhaps 20 million couples couple.

Globally, the human race is nearing 6 billion, including

about 2 billion adult couples. A 1992 study by the World Health Organization estimated that sexual intercourse occurs more than 100 million times a day—and that seems conservative. At any tick of the clock, hundreds of thousands of lovers around the planet are locked in passion, compelled by the urge driving all peoples in all centuries. Although it is unseen, it is a human activity of enormous significance.

The next time you and your lover sink into each other's arms, you will be part of a global pageant. And although you probably will be too absorbed to think about it, you will have vast multitudes of companions sharing the same joy and ardor.

Sex is nature at work. In this artificial world of offices and laws, money and machines, freeways and high-rises, it is a return to our basic biology.

We are designed to want each other. Our bodies generate the desire to find and keep a partner. We ceaselessly crave the most joyful experience two people can share.

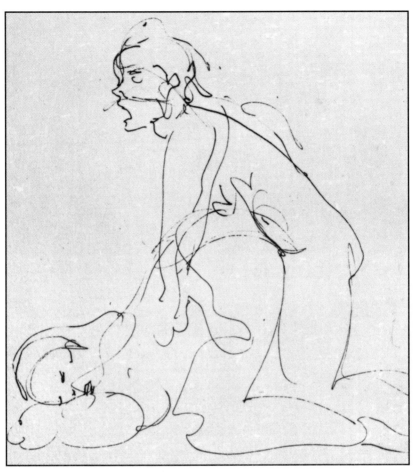

Leonor Fini. Ink sketch. © 1992 ARS, N.Y./SPADEM, Paris.

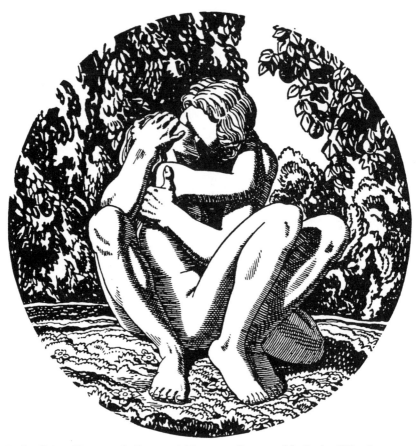

Rockwell Kent. Illustration for Boccaccio's *Decameron*. Courtesy of the Rockwell Kent Legacies.

And each was huddled in each other's love. . . .
　　　　　　—Louis Untermeyer, "Summer Storm"

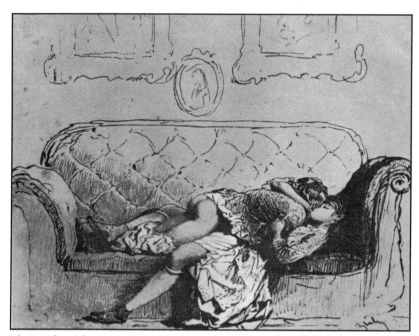

Above and next three pages. Hungarian-born artist Mihaly Zichy (1827-1906) created a series of 36 etchings collectively titled "Love," showing human affection from infancy to old age. This plate depicts a pair barely past puberty.

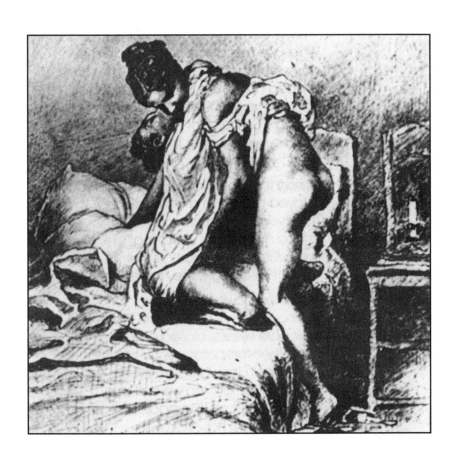

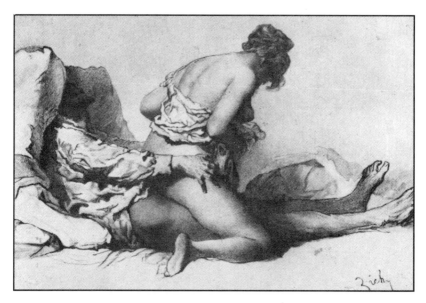

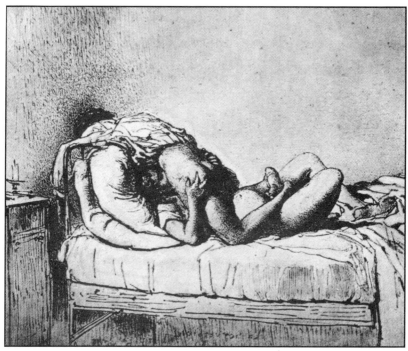

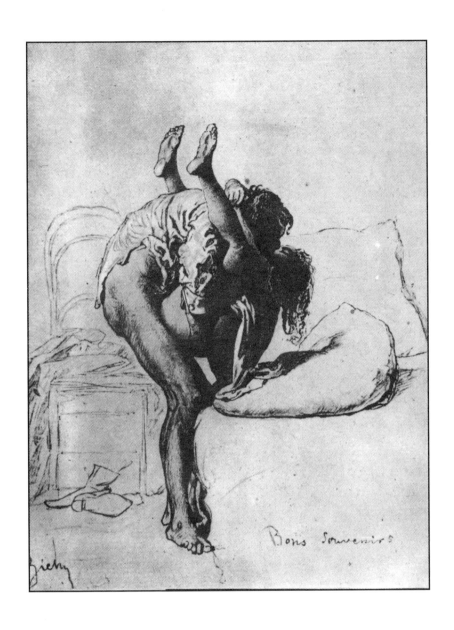

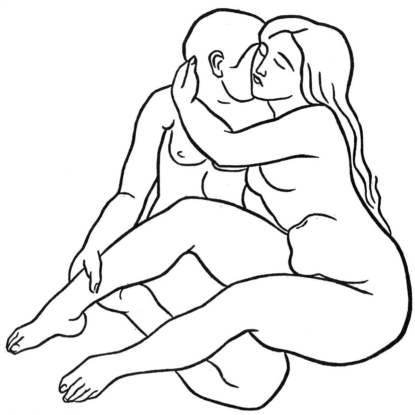

Aristide Maillol. Woodcut illustration for Ovid's *Art of Love.* © 1992 by ARS, N.Y./SPADEM, Paris.

Sex contains all, bodies, souls,

Meanings, proofs, purities, delicacies, results, promul-
gations, songs, commands, health, pride. . . .

All hopes, benefactions, bestowals, all the passions,
loves, beauties, delights of the earth.

—Walt Whitman, "A Woman Waits for Me," 1856

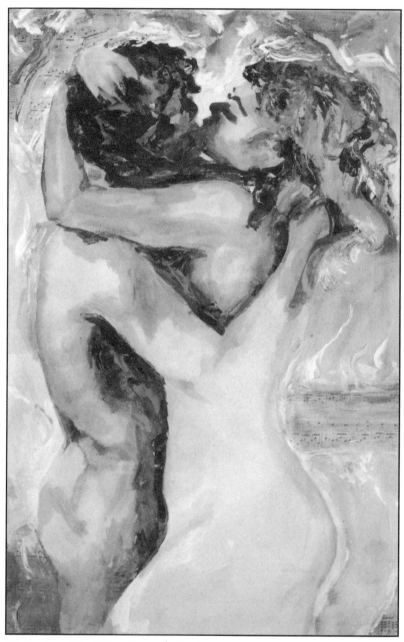

Silja Lahtinen. "The Willow Paints the Wind" (1988), acrylic, 30″ × 22″. Courtesy of the
artist.

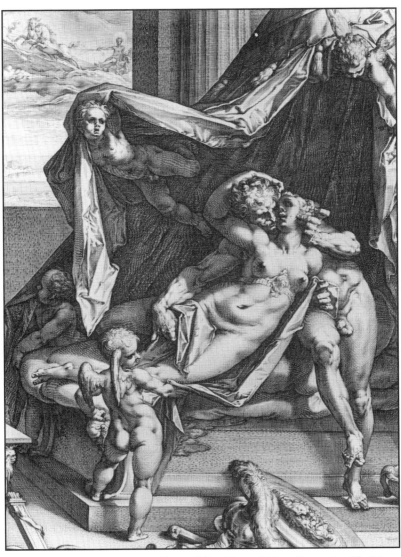

Hendrik Goltzius, after Spranger (16th c., 1588). "Mars and Venus," engraving. The Metropolitan Museum of Art, Harris Brisbane Dick Fund, 1953. [53.601.338 (63)]. All rights reserved. The Metropolitan Museum of Art.

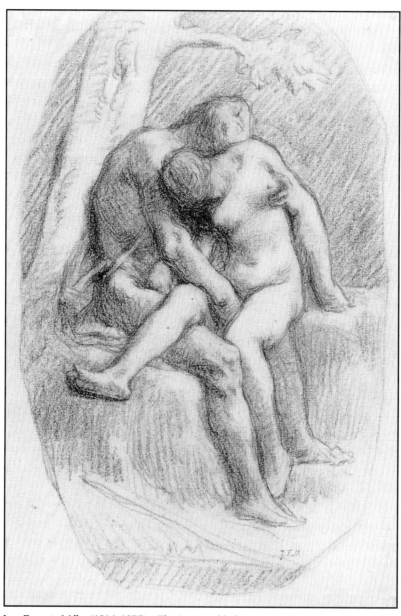

Jean-Francois Millet (1814–1875). "The Lovers," black crayon on tan wove paper, c. 1850, 32.5 × 22 cm., Charles Deering Collection. Photograph © 1992, The Art Institute of Chicago.

64

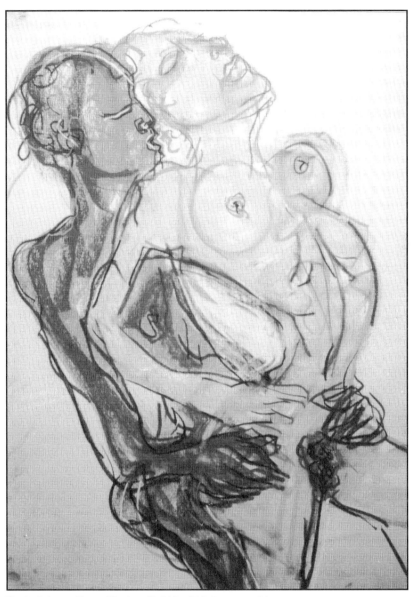

Phoebe Palmer. "Erotic #1" (pastel), 30″ × 22″. Courtesy of the artist.

Sex lies at the root of life, and we can never learn to rever-
ence life until we know how to understand sex.

—Havelock Ellis (1859–1939),
Studies in the Psychology of Sex

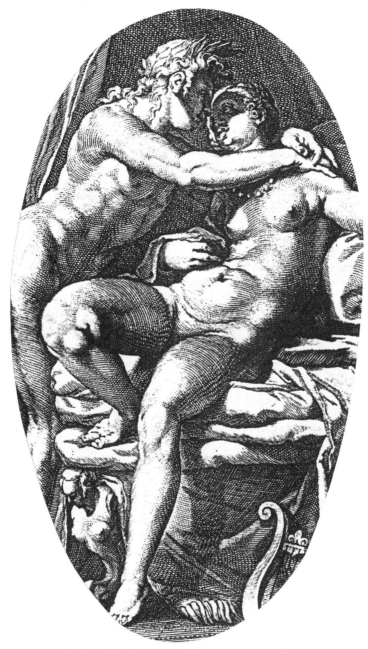

Hendrik Goltzius (1558–1617). "Phoebus and Clytie, or Love Triumphant," engraving.

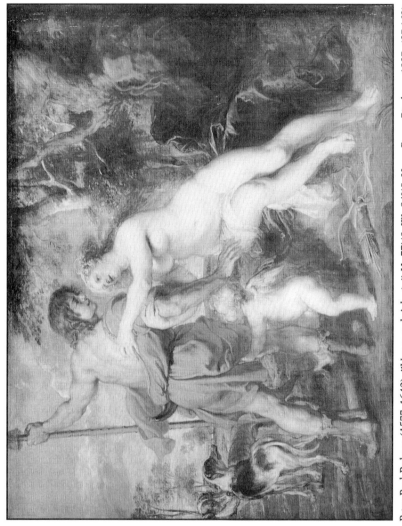

Peter Paul Rubens (1577–1640). "Venus and Adonis." H. 77½", W. 94⅞". Harry Payne Bingham, 1937. (37.162). All rights reserved. The Metropolitan Museum of Art.

68

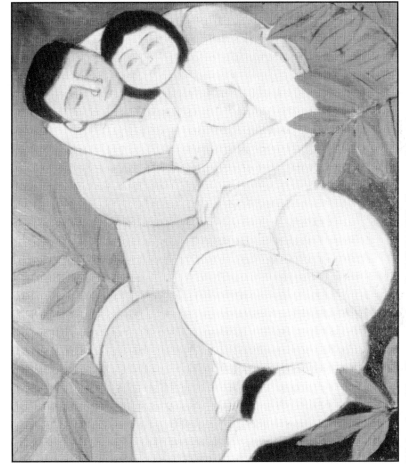

Bill Giacalone. "Two Figures with Leaves," oil (34" × 39"). Courtesy of the artist.

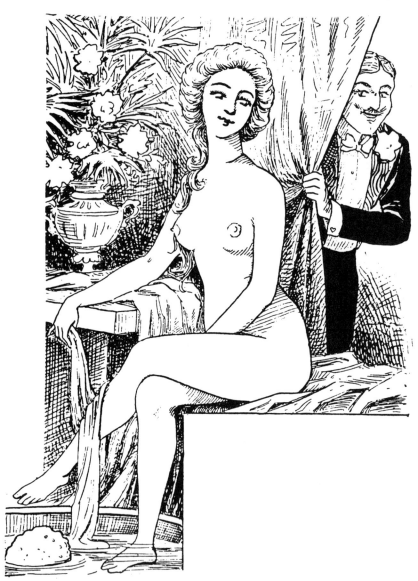

Above and next page. Nineteenth-century magazine illustrations.

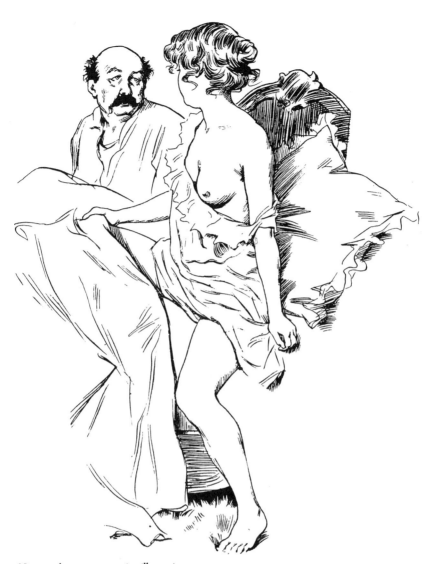

Nineteenth-century magazine illustration.

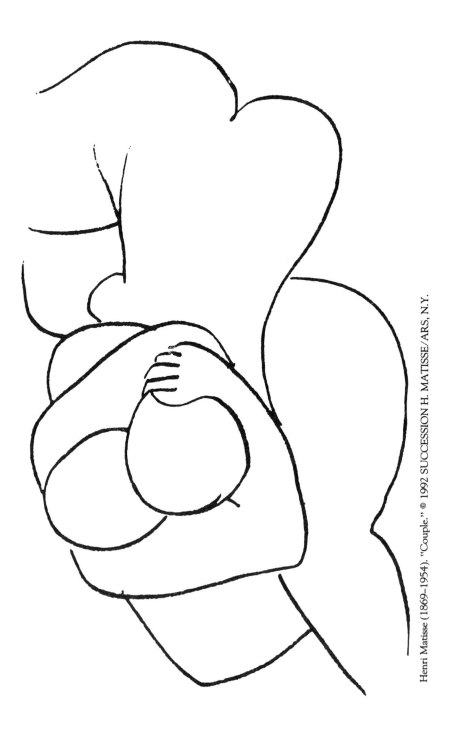

Henri Matisse (1869–1954). "Couple." © 1992 SUCCESSION H. MATISSE/ARS, N.Y.

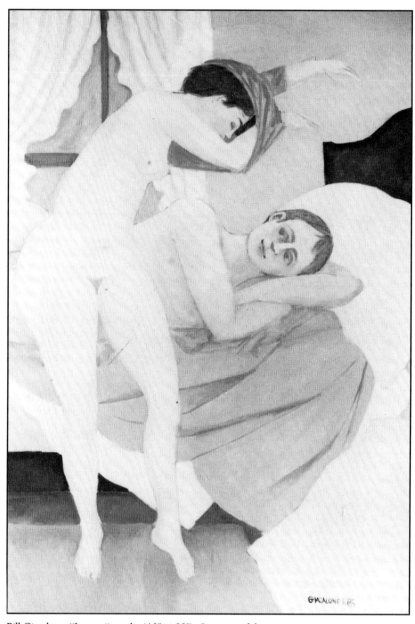

Bill Giacalone. "Lovers," acrylic (46″ × 66″). Courtesy of the artist.

THE SEXIEST ANIMAL

Sex is natural.

Lovemaking is as innate to people as eating, sleeping, breathing, growing, and all the other processes of life.

In fact, sex is more natural to humans than to virtually any other species.

Most creatures on the planet have slight sexuality, activated only in mating seasons. Many mammals function only once a year when the female is in heat—and even then they are limited. Fur obstructs their body contact. Rear-entry positions are impersonal. The females don't have orgasms. No other animal *enjoys* sex as much as people do. Evolution that gave humans a mighty brain and dextrous fingers also gave them the strongest sexuality on Earth.

Anthropologists and biologists generally concur that:

- Woman is the only female not bound by a period of heat. She is ready for sex every day of the year—which has made it natural for men and women to form permanent pairs, held together by the constant sharing of private pleasure. This pair-bonding has produced the family, hence the structure of societies.

- Women's vagina angle made face-to-face lovemaking natural for people, unlike the rear entry common to other species. This personalizes sex, making each partner special to the other.

75

It allows free range to kisses, caresses, hugs, and other joys of clasping each other.

- Woman may be the only female animal who has orgasms, which enhances her craving and gives her an incentive to keep the pair-bond strong.

- The loss of fur gave people bare skin—head-to-toe sensitivity to touch, increasing arousal.

- Men have the largest penises among primates—equipment for their expanded sexuality.

- Women's protruding breasts evidently evolved as sex lures. Protuberance isn't necessary for suckling. Female apes provide plenty of milk from flat, hair-hidden breasts. Presumably, prehistoric men were drawn to curvaceous women, impregnating them most often, and this natural selection magnified the bulge. Breasts have a sex role: they swell and nipples tighten during arousal. (By wearing brassieres, women unwittingly—or not-so-unwittingly—give their breasts the shape of sexual readiness.)

Spurred by all these biological enhancements, people copulate hundreds of times more than deer, or bears, or kangaroos—or even the legendary rabbits. (An exception is bonobos, dwarf chimpanzees, who mate so merrily that some researchers think they are the nearest evolutionary cousin of humans.)

"We are a species devoted to sex," anthropologist Helen Fisher wrote in *The Sex Contract*. "We talk about it, joke about it, read about it, dress for it, and perform it regularly. . . . Sexual traditions and behaviors saturate our lives."

Perhaps with a tinge of gender pride, Dr. Fisher attributes

this saturation to women, "the sex athletes of the primate world." She says the orgy occurs, "because the human female is capable of constant sexual arousal. She is physically able to make love every day of her adult life. She can copulate during pregnancy, and she can resume sexual activity shortly after having a child. She can make love whenever she pleases. This is extraordinary. No females of any other sexually reproducing species make love with such frequency. . . . In this respect she is unique among all other female creatures on earth. Women have lost their period of heat."

(Mark Twain expressed it well in *Letters From the Earth* when he noted that women are receptive to many "refreshments." Women are constantly "ready for action, and competent," Twain wrote. "As competent as the candlestick is to receive the candle. Competent every day, competent every night. Also, she *wants* that candle—yearns for it, longs for it, hankers after it, as commanded by the law of God in her heart.")

Dr. Fisher calls the pleasure bond between a man and woman "the sex contract"—an agreed sharing of lives "cemented by regular sex."

The need for a lover is fundamental to human life. Nobody should feel ashamed of it, or apologize for it.

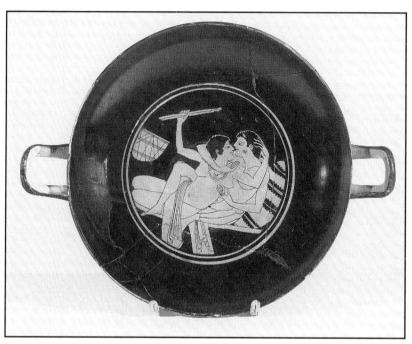

Red-figure kylix, Greek, Attic, ca. 510–500 B.C. Yale University Art Gallery, gift of Rebecca Darlington Stoddard.

As stolen love is pleasant to a man, so is it also to a woman.

—Ovid (43 B.C.–A.D. 17)

A lover's soul lives in the body of his mistress.

—Plutarch (ca. A.D. 46–119)

*Sweet in the heat of summer is cool water for one's thirst.
. . . But sweeter still two lovers when one mantle covers both.*

—Meleager, The Greek Anthology, 2nd century B.C.

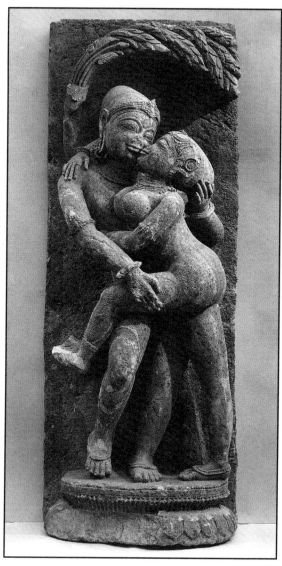

Indian sculpture, Orissa, 12th–13th century. Mithuna couple, stone. H. 6′. The Metropolitan Museum of Art, Florence Waterbury Fund, 1970. (1970.44). The Metropolitan Museum of Art.

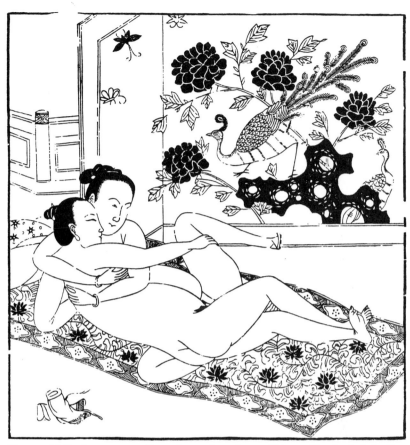

Above and following two pages. Illustrations and text from a Chinese pillow book dating from the late Ming Dynasty (1368–1644). *The Fragrant Flower: Classic Chinese Erotica in Art and Poetry*, trans. N. S. Wang and B. L. Wang (Buffalo, N.Y.: Prometheus Books, 1990).

(Coitus under Water in a Basin)

Carefully, silk robes are removed,
Together the perfumed waters are tried,
Paired like mandarin ducks frolicking in water,
Rumbling from the depths unceasing,
Warm and fragrant waves.
Spring mood is intense,
Disregarded is the ruined make-up,
Her pair of red lotus petals are reflected in the waves,
It is the moment of losing the souls,
Dew wetting the flower house.*

---

*orgasm—Trans.

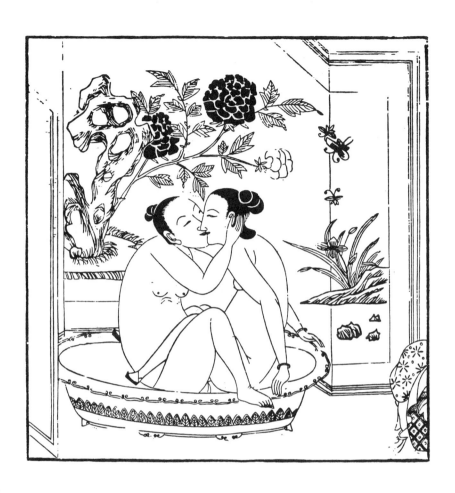

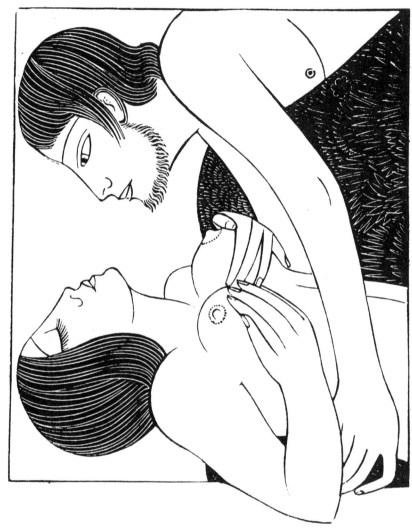

"I am my beloved's, and his desire is toward me." This line from the Bible's Song of Solomon was illustrated by ascetic and artist Eric Gill. Victoria and Albert Museum/Art Resource, N.Y.

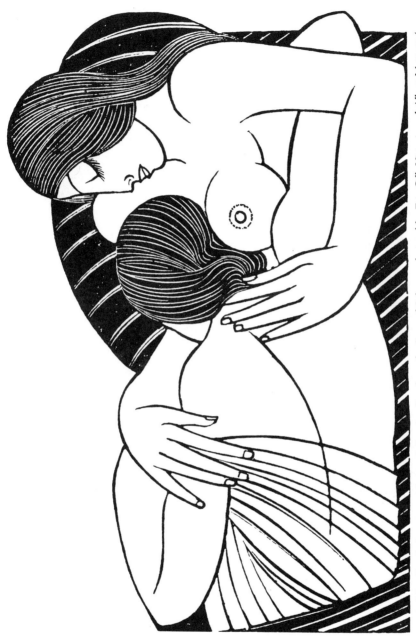

"He shall lie all night betwixt my breasts." Another line from the Song of Solomon depicted by Eric Gill. Victoria and Albert Museum/Art Resource, N.Y.

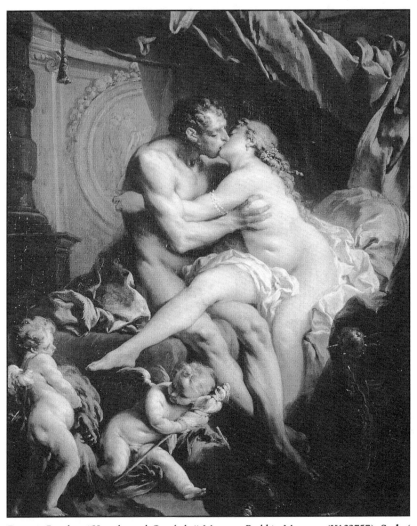

Francois Boucher. "Hercules and Omphale." Moscow: Pushkin Museum. (K102757). **Scala/ Art Resource, New York.**

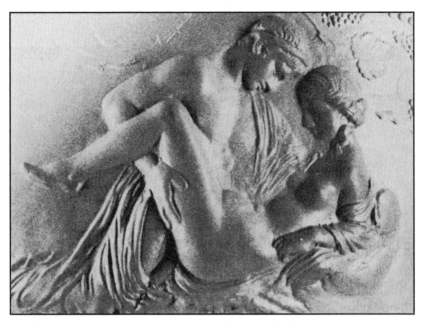

Vase figures by Marcus Perennius, first century B.C. Museo Archeologico, Arezzo.

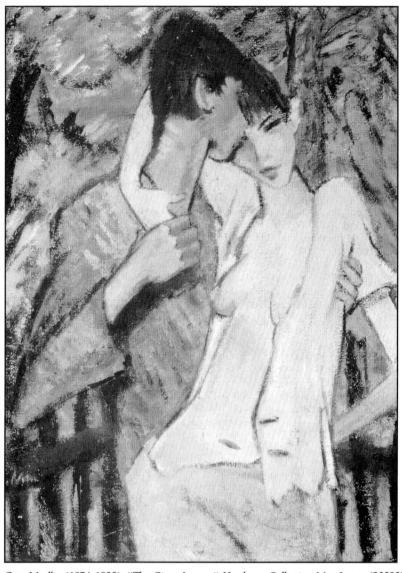

Otto Mueller (1874–1930). "The Gipsy Lovers." Hamburg: Collection Max Lutze. (20090). **Bridgeman/Art Resource, New York.**

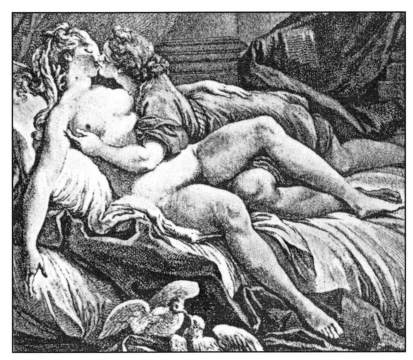

Vidal engraving, after Fragonard.

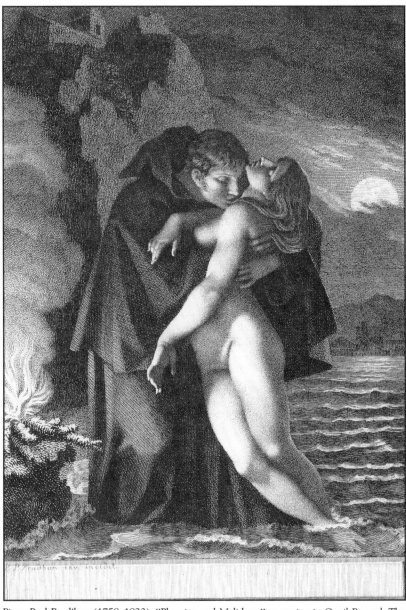

Pierre-Paul Prud'hon (1758–1823). "Phrosine and Melidore," engraving in *Gentil Bernard*. The Metropolitan Museum of Art, Harris Brisbane Dick Fund, 1938 (38.38.4). All rights reserved. The Metropolitan Museum of Art.

90

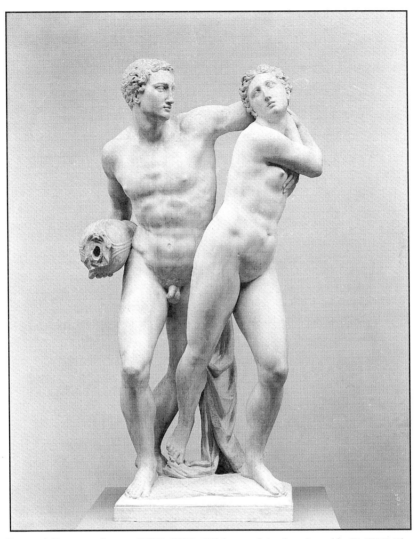

Battista di Domenico Lorenzi (1527?–1594). "Alpheus and Arethusa," marble. H. 58¾". The Metropolitan Museum of Art, Fletcher Fund, 1940 (40.33). All rights reserved. The Metropolitan Museum of Art.

How beautiful are thy feet with shoes, O prince's daughter! The joints of thy thighs are like jewels, the work of the hands of a cunning workman. . . .

Thy navel is like a round goblet, which wanteth not liquor. Thy belly is like a heap of wheat set about with lilies. . . .

Thy two breasts are like two young roes that are twins. Thy neck is as a tower of ivory.

Thine eyes are like the fishpools in Heshbon. . . .

How fair and how pleasant art thou, O love, for delights! . . .

—The Song of Solomon, 7

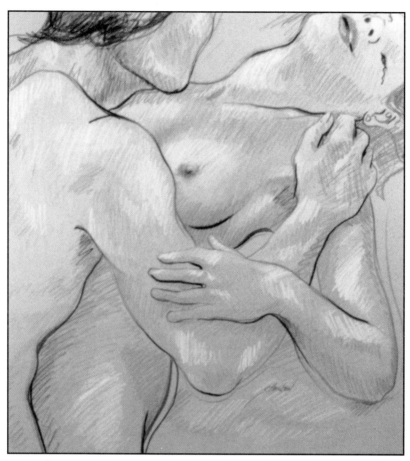

Steven Hamilton. "Whispers," color pencil on board (18″ × 17″). © 1990 Steven Hamilton. Courtesy of the artist.

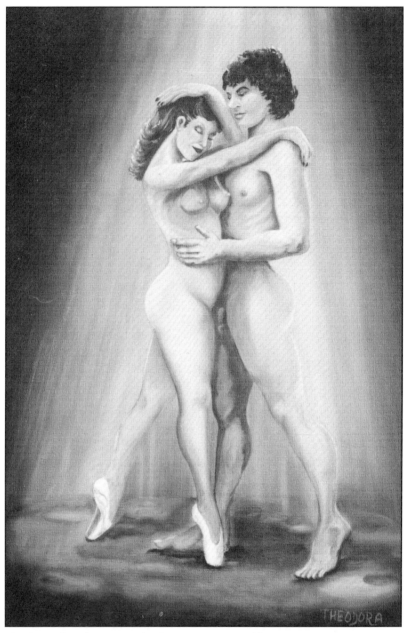

Theodora Cislo. "The Dance," oil (16″ × 20″). Courtesy of the artist.

Sexuality is the lyricism of the masses.
　　　　　—Charles Baudelaire, *Intimate Journal*

Rare are they who prefer virtue to the pleasures of sex.
　　　　　—Confucius

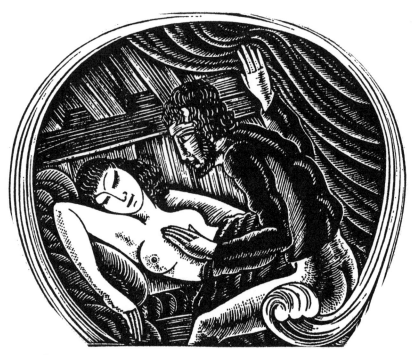

Eric Gill. "Woman Asleep," engraving (1936). Victoria and Albert Museum/Art Resource, N.Y.

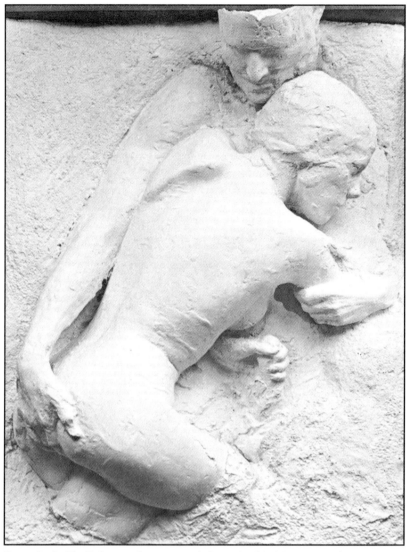

George Segal. "The Embrace," plaster casting. © George Segal/VAGA, New York, 1992.

CRUEL TABOOS

Humankind has a streak of madness that produces self-inflicted wounds. Senseless suffering fills history: hideous wars, the Inquisition, human sacrifice, Hiroshima, Auschwitz, death squads, Jonestown.

Similarly, sex has been twisted into a topic of torment. Instead of accepting the libido for what it is—a healthy blessing of nature—many cultures have branded sex as "dirty," "sinful," and "filthy," tolerating it only under confined conditions. Guilt, shame, fear, and punishment have been inflicted on multitudes of men and women.

The Old Testament mandated that adulterers "shall surely be put to death," by stoning or by fire. (The fact that Solomon had 700 wives and 300 concubines, and "loved many foreign women," didn't soften this death penalty.) The Koran commands that unwed Muslim lovers shall be stoned to death or flogged. (The Koran allows each man four wives and various concubines, and promises him a heaven full of female houri nymphs—but that doesn't alter the grim punishment.) In ancient China, unmarried lovers faced mutilation for the man and drowning for the woman. In Vietnam, the traditional punishment for women who strayed was to be trampled by a trained elephant.

Religious obsession against sex reached bizarre heights in the 1500s, when the Inquisition tortured thousands of women into confessing they were witches who copulated with Satan—and then burned them alive for it. In the 1600s, when Puritans ruled England, adultery by married people was punishable by death, while sex between singles drew prison terms. In Puritan New England, unmarried lovers were flogged, locked in public pillories, or forced to slink about in shame wearing "the scarlet letter," an A for adultery.

The rise of democracy and human rights slowly erased this cruelty in the Western world. "The pursuit of happiness" became legitimate. Finally in the 20th century, most Western nations abandoned laws that once threw lovers into cells.

But taboos still mar many lands. Some Muslim societies force women to cloak themselves to the eyes. Death by stoning for unmarried lovers is still commanded in Pakistan, the United Arab Emirates, and elsewhere. In Saudi Arabia, a teenage princess and her lover were executed in public in 1977 for the crime of making love. In Iran, women are segregated from public life, and morality patrols hunt those who allow a lock of hair to escape from their shrouds. In some African cultures, women's clitorises are amputated or their vaginas sewn shut, to keep them "pure."

Even in modern America, religious extremists still seek to ban television programs that "condone sex," to censor library books, and to halt sex education in schools. Catholic leaders still forbid 50 million Americans to use birth-control devices. Ex-nun Patricia Hussey said in her book *No Turning Back* (1990): "The church really hates the idea of people having sex for fun. . . . There is something prurient and dishonest about the church's loathing for the body." Even in the liberal-minded Episcopal faith, when Bishop John Spong proposed blessing unmarried couples in 1988, he was denounced by angry church-men and received death threats. When a Presbyterian commission declared in 1991, "We affirm the goodness of sexual intimacy," and sought to change church policy about sex, it was overwhelmingly rejected by the Presbyterian national assembly.

Why is there such revulsion to simple biology? Americans don't object to "slasher" movies in which fiends decapitate teenagers, or "Rambo" films filled with slaughter. Killing is modern entertainment, but love is less acceptable. In the words of a popular song: "Bullets fly like popcorn on the screen, recommended wholesome, nice, and clean. Making love's the thing that can't be seen. Why?"

As the contents of this book reveal, master artists through the centuries have depicted men and women in their moments of deepest intimacy. Some of this art was done in secret, kept in private sketchbooks not discovered until after the artists' death. Other works were preserved in private collections by the wealthy—or, ironically, by the church. Common people caught looking at such pictures risked imprisonment.

It was not until the postwar era in America that crusaders against censorship finally won court rulings allowing the hidden paintings and sketches to emerge. Even so, part of the populace still regards sex as a shameful topic to be concealed. Certain legislators still advocate laws that would send you to jail for looking at this book. So the struggle goes on and on, evolving but never ceasing.

Aversion to sex seems irrational. Anatole France wrote, "Of all the sexual aberrations, chastity is the strangest." Television commentator Phil Donahue summed it up well in his book, *The Human Animal*:

101

"How do we play this cruel joke on ourselves? How does the human mind take one of our greatest joys—a pleasure we're better equipped to enjoy than any other animal—and transform it into one of our greatest guilts?"

Only a diabolical mind could do this, he said—the human mind.

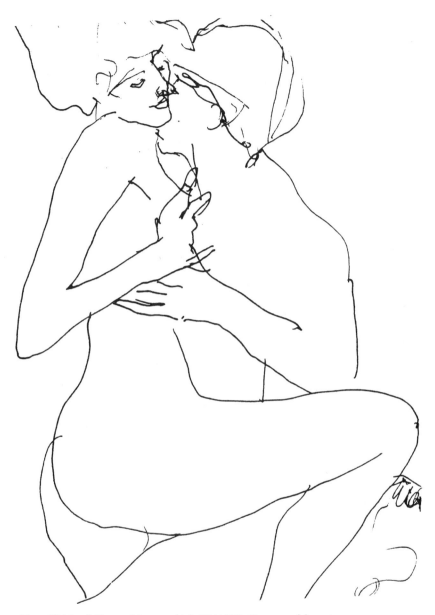

Harry Weisburd. "Lovers I," pen and ink (9″ × 12″). Courtesy of the artist.

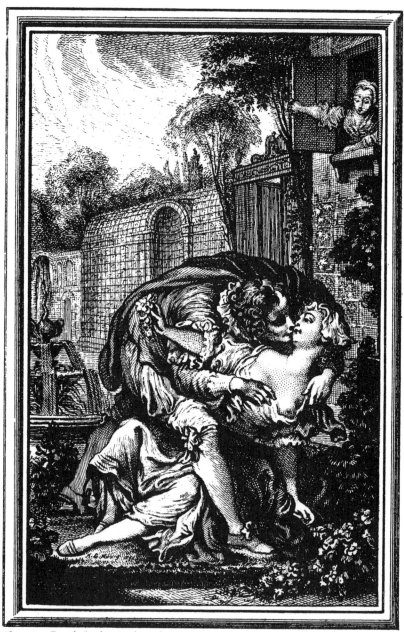

"Love in a French Garden," eighteenth-century print.

License my roving hands, and let them go,
Before, behind, between, above, below.
　　　　—John Donne, "To His Mistress Going to Bed"

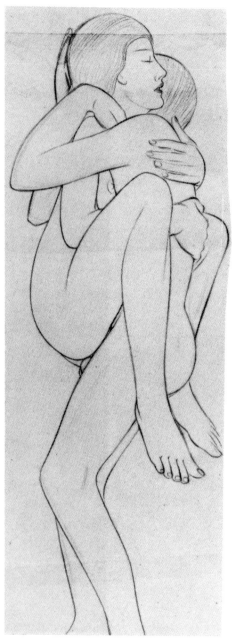

Eric Gill. Colored drawing. Victoria and Albert
Museum/Art Resource, N.Y.

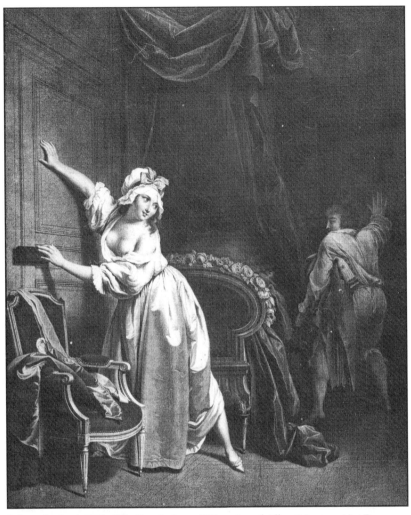

Etching after Louis Boilly, "The Favorite Lover." **Victoria and Albert Museum / Art Resource, N.Y.**

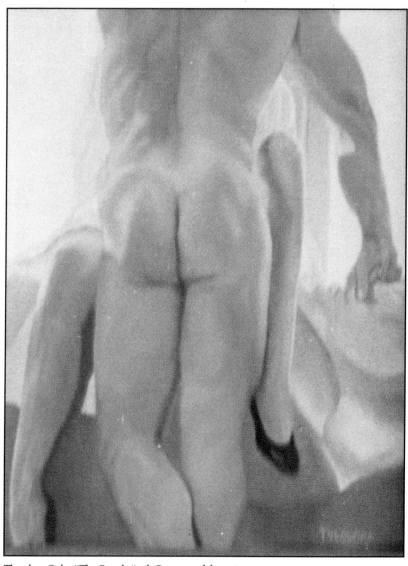

Theodora Cislo. "The Couple," oil. Courtesy of the artist.

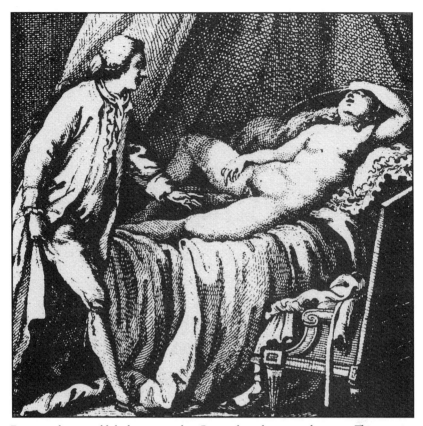

Erotic novels were published anonymously in Paris in the early nineteenth century. This engraving is from the novel *Felicia*, ca. 1800.

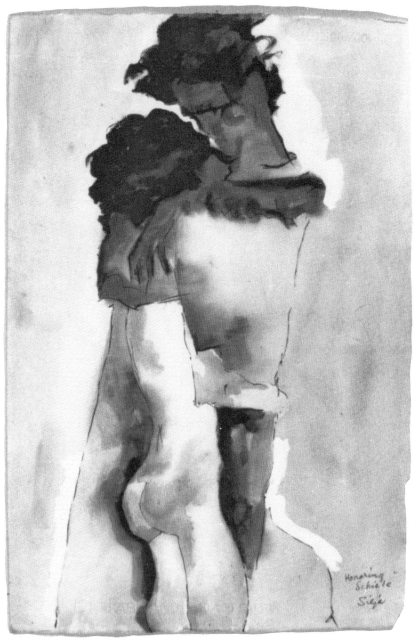

Silja Lahtinen. "Lovers" (1985), acrylic, watercolor, gouache on Fabriano, 22″ × 15″. Courtesy of the artist.

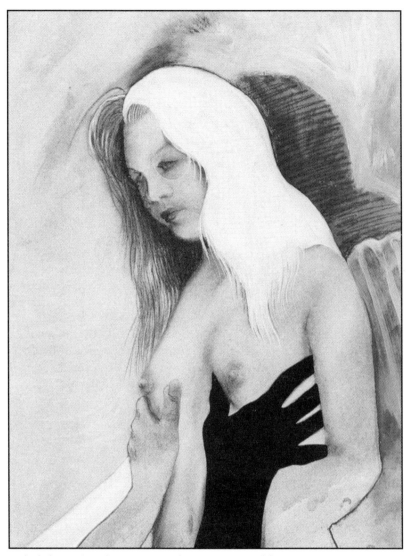

Michael Florian Jilg. "Blue Movie," pastel, gesso. Courtesy of the artist.

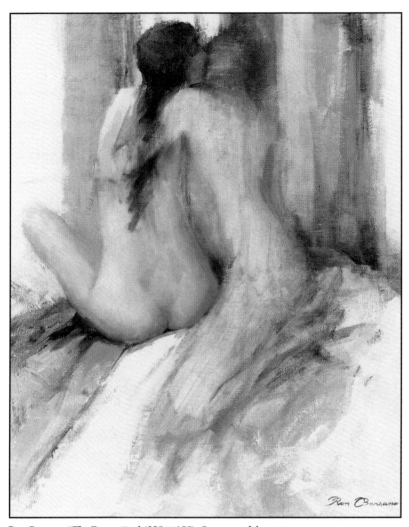

Ron Barsano. "The Dream," oil (22″ × 18″). Courtesy of the artist.

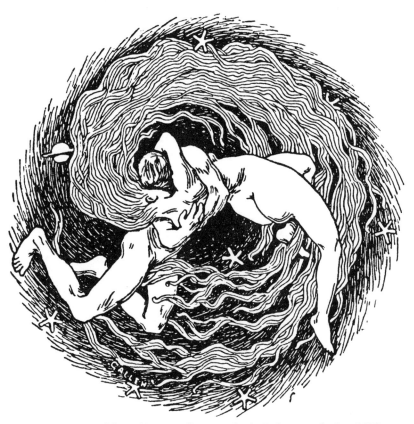

Axel Gallen-Kallela (1865–1931). Illustration for the Berlin quarterly, *Pan* (1895).

Come, my Celia, let us prove, while we can, the sports of love.

—Ben Jonson, *Volpone* (1605)

On his neck her yoking arms she throws:
She sinketh down, still hanging by his neck,
He on her belly falls, she on her back.
Now is she in the very lists of love,
Her champion mounted for the hot encounter:
All is imaginary she doth prove,
He will not manage her, although he mount her.

—Shakespeare, *Venus and Adonis*

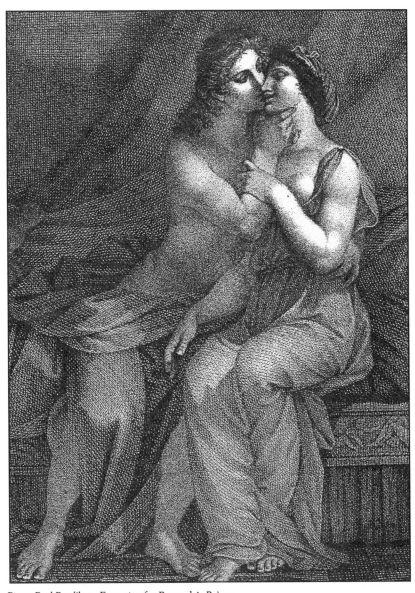

Pierre-Paul Prud'hon. Engraving for Bernarde's *Poèmes*.

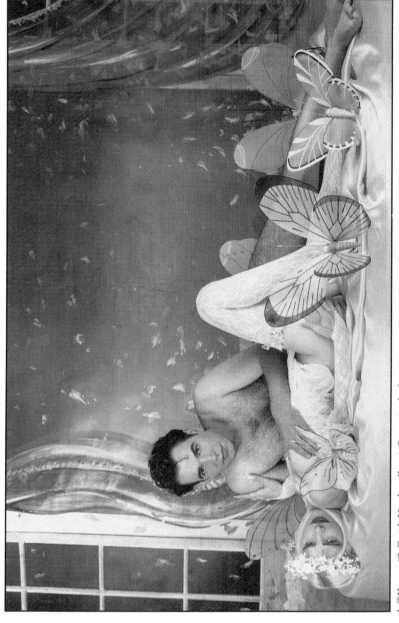

Jeff Koons. "Jeff with Hand on Ilona's Breast," oil inks on canvas. Copyright © Jeff Koons. Courtesy of the artist.

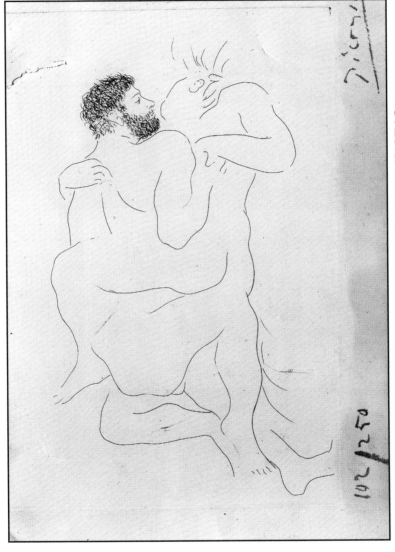

Pablo Picasso. "A Man and a Woman" (1927). Private collection. © 1992, ARS, N.Y./SPADEM, Paris.

117

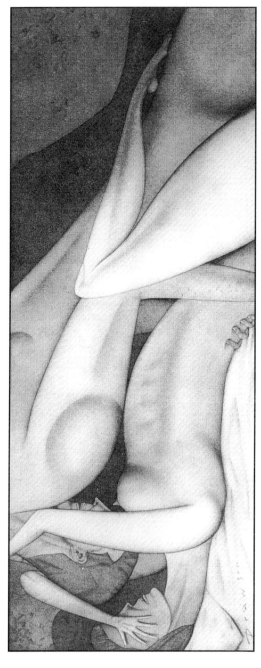

Blair Drawson. "You and Me," watercolor (18½″ × 7¼″). Courtesy of the artist.

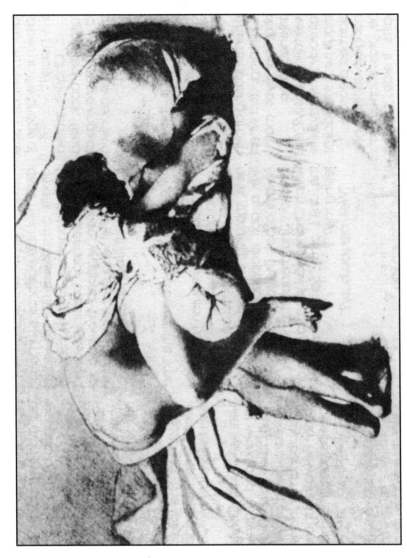

Mihaly Zichy. Another etching in his "Love" series.

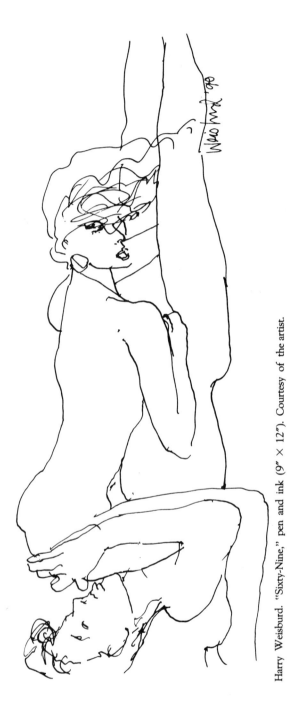

Harry Weisburd. "Sixty-Nine," pen and ink (9" × 12"). Courtesy of the artist.

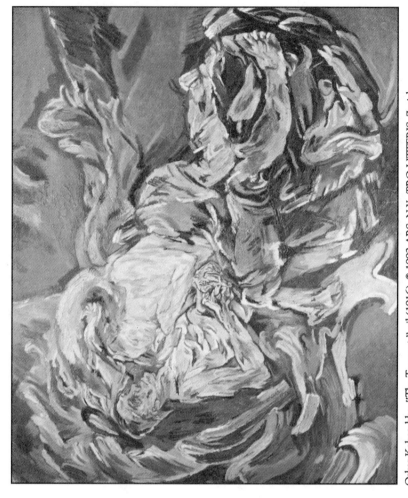

THE TWOSQUARE THING

For sheer contentment and inner peace, nothing is better than the bond of a loving couple who make each other happy in bed. A good sex life heals the frustrations of the daily world.

Austrian painter Oskar Kokoschka (1886–1980) once painted himself and his lover nestling in bed, unfazed by the jagged torments around them. The Nazis purged Kokoschka's work as "degenerate"—but the world holds a different opinion. Art critic John Canaday, in a Metropolitan Museum of Art seminar series, has described the self-portrait as showing "that human love is the sustaining miracle of goodness in the confusion and malevolence of life. The figures are 'ugly' because they must participate in life; they are worn by it. They have not escaped from life, they have found a refuge within it."

This refuge gives couples a shared security that can be seen in their faces. James Thurber, in *One Is a Wanderer*, called the relationship "a twosquare thing." Anne Morrow Lindbergh, in *Gift from the Sea*, called such pairs a "double sunrise" seashell with two snug-fitting halves.

The bond is precious—but it is elusive and fragile. The twosquare thing is difficult to find, and more difficult to maintain. A discouraging number of relationships flounder and disintegrate. Half of U.S. marriages end in divorce. Many others decline into boredom or strife. Worst of all, some become violent: more than 2,000 Americans kill their mates each year, and thousands of beatings occur.

Still, despite all the trouble, men and women need each other, and are driven by a compulsion to attain fulfillment. Scholar Morton Hunt has argued that the high divorce rate "reflects not so much the failure of love as the determination of people not to live without it." A good bond is a goal worth everyone's relentless pursuit. Searching for the right partner, then working endlessly to maintain the partnership, can bring a priceless reward.

In today's evolving society, many pairs seek "the sustaining miracle" in togetherness outside marriage. Whatever the arrangement, sex is nature's binding force cementing couples. The phrase "making love" has a double meaning: through good sex, men and women generate love. And it makes their lives rich.

This force increasingly is being liberated. The "sexual revolution" is real. Profound changes have occurred within the life-span of mature Americans. Consider:

• Nude lovemaking is common in today's R-rated movies, and bare bodies abound in magazines—but such depictions caused police raids and jail sentences a generation ago. Even describing sex in words was a crime under old censorship laws.

• About 3 million unmarried American couples now live together openly, with little disapproval by families or land-lords—yet such cohabitation was unthinkable in the 1950s, often bringing prosecution.

• Birth-control pills and condoms are dispensed to high school students now—but birth-control pioneers were jailed early in this century, and contraception remained a crime in

124

Catholic Massachusetts until a landmark 1972 Supreme Court ruling.

• Homosexuals are generally accepted today—but gays were sentenced to prison under biblical "sodomy" laws until the 1970s. In fact, oral sex was a crime even for married couples in most states.

A wave of personal freedom has swept through America since World War II, overcoming centuries of shame and suppression. Censors and religious extremists resisted—and still resist—each step, but the liberation tide left them at the fringe. The transformation reflects a profound change of attitude in Western culture.

However, while many strictures have faded, one code survives: the belief that fidelity is best between committed couples. The emotional bond between lovers is rooted deep in the nature of people, and pain always results when one partner breaches the exclusivity. It's true that some people practice casual sex or multiple relationships—which is their privilege—but the majority still believes in the romantic ideal, the twosquare thing, the double sunrise. No matter how often this ideal is shattered, the belief endures like a religious tenet.

Amid the world's chaos and sham, amid all the unreason and greed, it isn't easy to find something to trust. But faith can be placed in the human instinct to mate. Never stop believing in the bond between a man and a woman. Never stop believing that it can be a treasure.

When two people are right for each other, sex is beautiful.

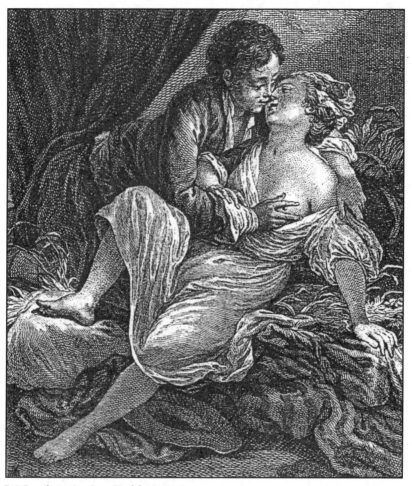

P-A Beaudoin. "Les Soins Tardifs," engraving.

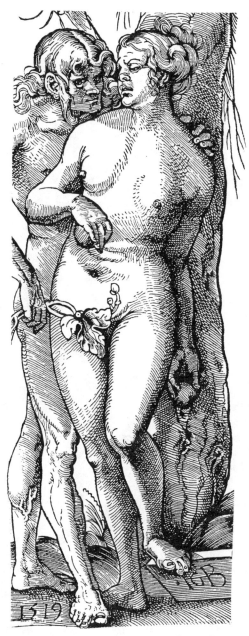

Hans Baldung-Grien (1484–1545). "Adam and Eve," engraving.

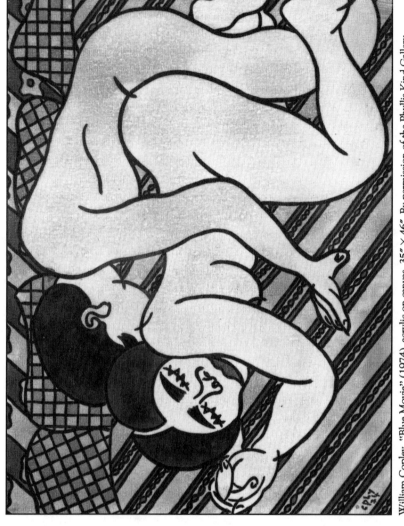

William Copley. "Blue Movie" (1974), acrylic on canvas, 35" × 46". By permission of the Phyllis Kind Gallery.

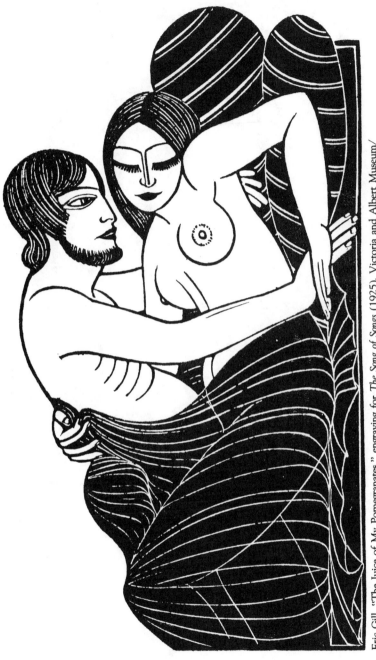

Eric Gill. "The Juice of My Pomegranates," engraving for *The Song of Songs* (1925). Victoria and Albert Museum/ Art Resource, N.Y.

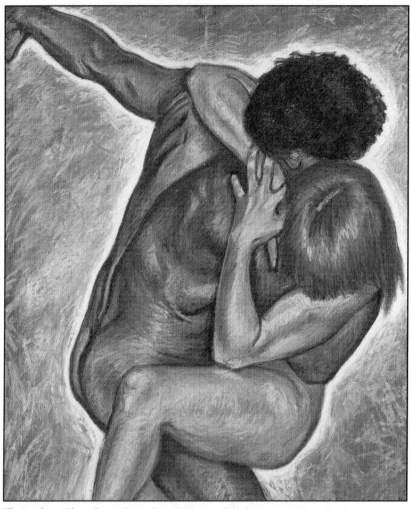

Elli Crocker. "Please Don't Go #15" (1988), mixed media/paper, 48″ × 42″. By permission of the artist.

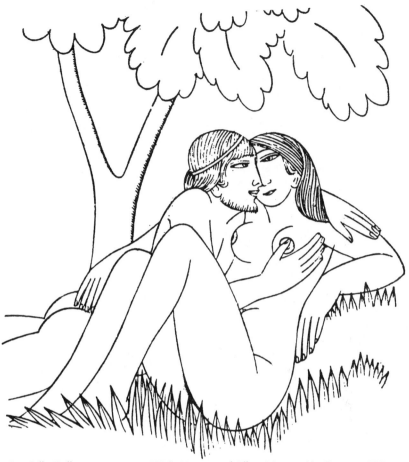

Eric Gill. "Dalliance," engraving (1926). Victoria and Albert Museum/Art Resource, N.Y.

And they were both naked, the man and his wife, and were not ashamed.

—Genesis 2

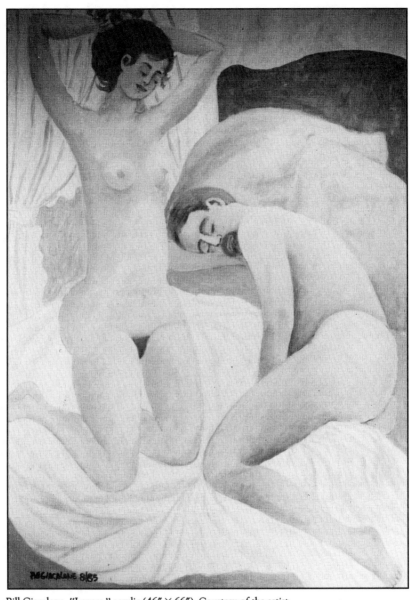

Bill Giacalone. "Lovers," acrylic (46″ × 66″). Courtesy of the artist.

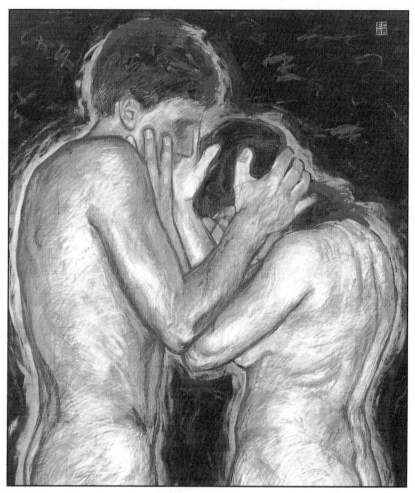

Elli Crocker. "Please Don't Go #14" (1988), mixed media/paper, 48″ × 42″. By permission of the artist.

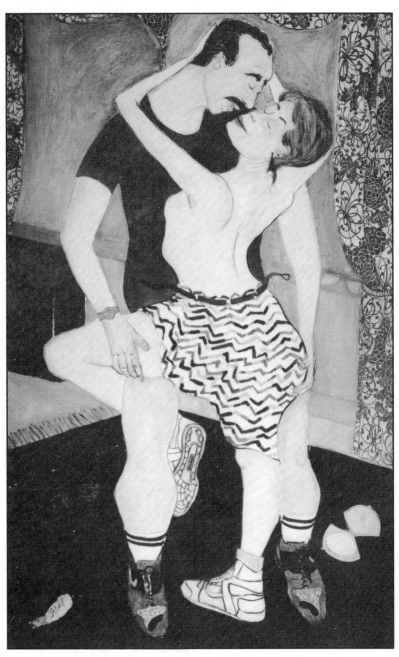

Phoebe Palmer. "Success of Modern Footwear," oil (5′ × 3′). Courtesy of the artist.

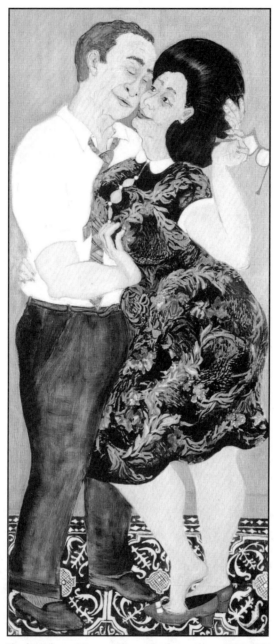

Phoebe Palmer. "Steamy Glasses," oil on canvas, 1988 (36″
× 84″). Courtesy of the artist.

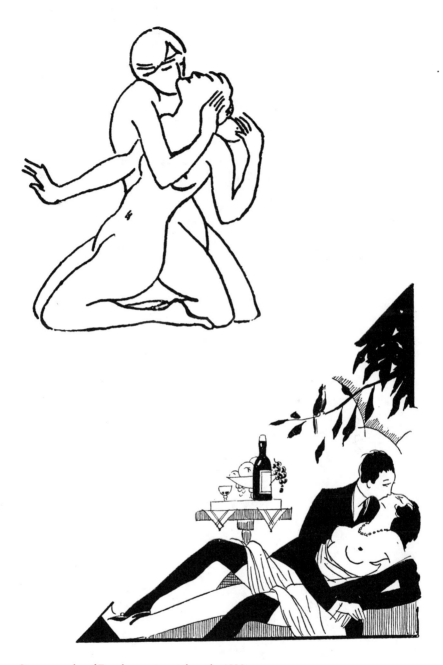

Some examples of French magazine art from the 1920s.

. . . my God after that long kiss I near lost my breath yes he
said I was a flower of the mountain yes so we are flowers
all a womans body yes . . . and then I asked him with my
eyes to ask again yes and then he asked me would I yes to
say yes my mountain flower and first I put my arms around
him yes and drew him down to me so he could feel my
breasts all perfume yes and his heart was going like mad
and yes I said yes I will yes.

—Molly Bloom in *Ulysses*, James Joyce
© 1990, Vintage Press

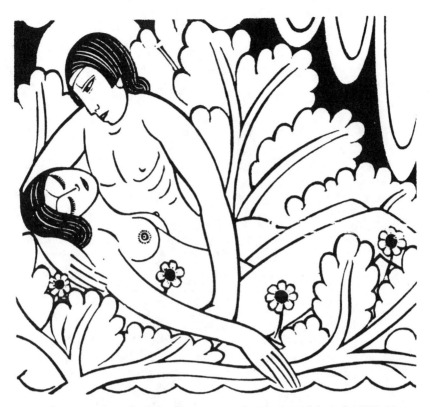

Eric Gill. "Our Bed Is All of Flowers," engraving for *The Song of the Soul* (1927). Victoria and Albert Museum/Art Resource, N.Y.

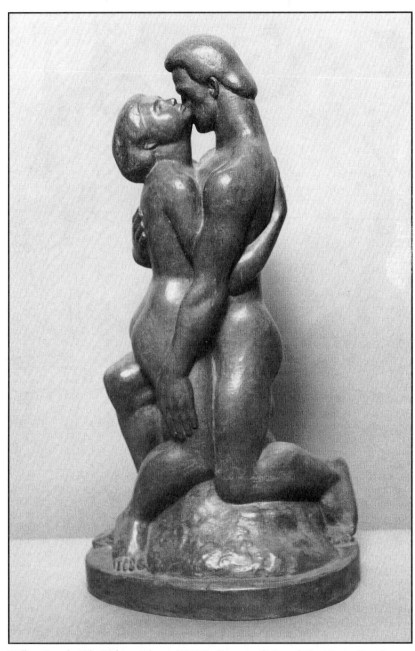

William Zorach. "The Embrace," bronze (1933). Courtesy of Mr. and Mrs. Tessim Zorach.

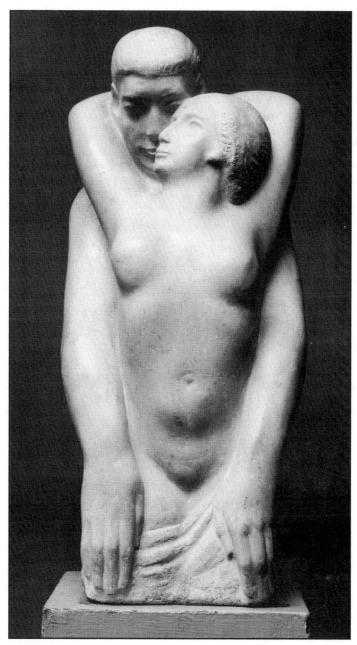

William Zorach. "Love" (1959), marble, 24″ h. Private collection.

Somewhere there waiteth in this world of ours
    For one lone soul another lonely soul,
Each choosing each through all the weary hours,
    And meeting strangely at one sudden goal,
Then blend they, like green leaves with golden flowers,
    Into one beautiful and perfect whole;
And life's long night is ended, and the way
    Lies open onward to eternal day.
                —Edwin Arnold (1832–1904),
                 "Somewhere There Waiteth"

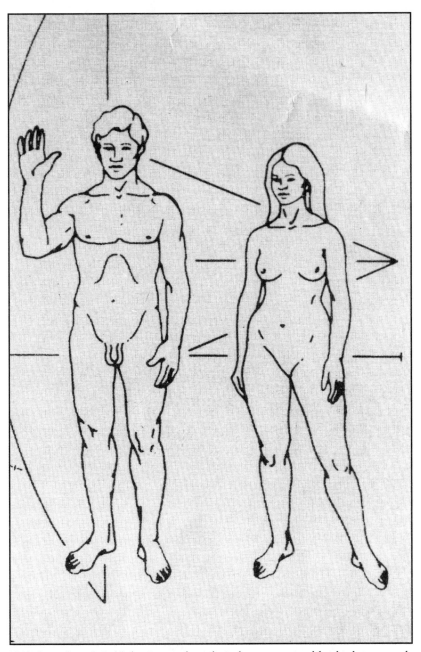

Natural, unashamed, and belonging together—that's the tone conveyed by this human couple
etched on the Pioneer 10 and 11 space probes as part of the greeting to any aliens the craft
may encounter billions of miles from Earth. Courtesy of the National Aeronautics and Space
Administration.

INDEX OF ARTISTS